How to Create the

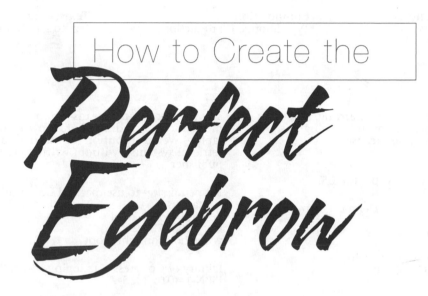

Perfect Eyebrow

Victoria Bush

THOMSON

™

DELMAR LEARNING

Australia Canada Mexico Singapore Spain United Kingdom United States

THOMSON

DELMAR LEARNING

How to Create the Perfect Eyebrow
Victoria Bush

MILADY STAFF

President:
Dawn Gerrain

Director of Editorial:
Sherry Gomoll

Acquisitions Editor:
Stephen G. Smith

Developmental Editor:
Judy Aubrey Roberts

Editorial Assistant:
Courtney VanAuskas

Director of Production:
Wendy A. Troeger

Production Editor:
Eileen M. Clawson

Production Assistant:
Erica R. Seeley

Composition:
Type Shoppe II Productions

Marketing Specialist:
Sandra Bruce

Marketing Coordinator:
Kasmira Koniszewski

Cover Design:
Dutton and Sherman Design

Text Design:
Liz Kodela Graphic Design

Library of Congress Cataloging-in-Publication Data
ISBN 1-4018-3335-7

NOTICE TO THE READER

I dedicate this book to my husband Frank and my children, Stephanie, and Rachel, who have encouraged, supported, and loved me throughout this project. You are the lights of my life, and I love you so much.

I give special thanks to Kathleen Weiss for her time and expertise in editing the book. Her tireless effort has made it the best it can be. I thank Rosemarie Kovacs, who dedicated so much time and effort in helping to make Adriel, Inc. a successful endeavor.

I also thank other members of my family for their support and love: my parents, Victor and Rosemarie; Frank's parents, Barney and Ginny; Rich; Kathy; Larry; Andrew; Ryan; Alex; Andy; Sherri; Laura; Dave; Kate; Kinsey; Robert; and Irene.

Last, I thank the Petruccelli family, Rose Marie Beauchemin, Rhonda Thomson, Tony Del Verme, Kristin Machesky, Israel Gonzalez, Tweezerman Corporation, and Bianco Brothers.

—Victoria Bush

Contents

Preface ix

CHAPTER 1 – The Art and Science of Creating Beautiful, Symmetrical Eyebrows 1

CHAPTER 2 – The Study of the Facial Zones. 11

CHAPTER 3 – The Study of the Geometric Face Shapes 19

CHAPTER 4 – The Study of Eye Set 29

CHAPTER 5 – Assessing the Facial Features 35

CHAPTER 6 – Assessing the Eyebrow 45

CHAPTER 7 – Rules of Proper Eyebrow Management 55

CHAPTER 8 – Corrective Techniques to the Eyebrow to Enhance
the Features of the Face 67

CHAPTER 9 – Eyebrow Design Methods 77

CHAPTER 10 – Performing Eyebrow Design and Enhancement 83

CHAPTER 11 – Hair Removal for the Eyebrows 101

CHAPTER 12 – Other Eyebrow Enhancement Services 125

CHAPTER 13 - Case Studies: Eyebrow Design in Practice 133

Appendix A: Answers to Chapter Quizzes 159

Appendix B: Resource Directory 163

Index 169

Perhaps more has been written recently about the quiet little hairs above the eyes than any other feature of the face. Newspaper articles, magazine articles, and books written by makeup artists all add to this proliferation of "brow talk." This extensive print coverage is not limited to beauty or fashion magazines or small local newspapers. Mainstream media giants have added to the media frenzy regarding this topic as well. Front page news articles on the subject of eyebrows have been printed in both *The Wall Street Journal* and *USA Today*. In addition, talk shows such as "Oprah" and "Good Morning America" have invited brow experts to share their knowledge with the public. This expansive media coverage indicates that the topic is not only of importance to many people but also that there is a tremendous potential for profit in becoming an eyebrow expert.

How to Create the Perfect Eyebrow is written for students in all disciplines in the beauty industry and for licensed, practicing beauty professionals. The list of beauty industry disciplines includes such areas of specialization as cosmetology, esthetics, makeup, temporary hair removal, electrology, and permanent makeup. The concepts set forth in this book are universal and are, therefore, applicable in every country in the world. Anyone, anywhere, who has an interest in the beauty industry will profit greatly from its unique contents.

Why this Book Was Written— Trends and a Void

The latest trends in the market show an increased demand by the consumer for expertise in eyebrow enhancement. According to *USA Today* (Giving Eyebrows a New Lift: Brow Boutiques Spreading Coast to Coast, July 13, 2000), "These days, eyebrow stylists are on America's most wanted list . . . chic 'brow boutiques' are spreading from the West and East coasts to Miami, Dallas, and beyond."

InStyle, *Cosmopolitan*, *Allure*, and other popular consumer magazines consistently print articles about eyebrows. *Les Nouvelles Esthetiques*, *Dermascope*, *Skin, Inc.*, *Modern Salon*, and other important professional industry publications also consistently maintain that the eyebrows are one of the most important aspects of overall beauty. The ongoing flow of information is proof that the focus on eyebrows is here to stay and will intensify as more people clamor to learn how to optimally perform this service.

It is this ongoing trend in the market, coupled with the lack of an existing authoritative resource on the subject, that has created the need for *How to Create the Perfect Eyebrow*.

How this Book Was Written—Research and Hands-on Experience

How to Create the Perfect Eyebrow was written following years of experience and intense research. The research began with a thorough study of the face shapes, facial features, and longstanding rules of eyebrow enhancement. Next, the work of makeup artists and other beauty professionals was examined to find where the experts agreed and where they disagreed with respect to these areas of study. Finding that there was, indeed, a great deal of agreement and disagreement on much of the subject matter lead to further study and a desire to present the differing theories to students and beauty professionals for further evaluation and learning.

One example of a subject about which there are varying opinions is the study of face shapes. In Chapter 3, the different face shape theories are introduced and shown in the various ways they are taught. No one technique is put forth as the correct way. Instead, the various options are presented, which allows the beauty professional to choose his or her preference based on that person's expanded knowledge and experience.

Our team of makeup artists put the theories and rules to the test and performed thousands of eyebrow makeovers at salon trade shows, salon distributor shows, and in private consultations. Our company, on invitation from Tweezerman Corporation, began performing eyebrow makeovers at the International Beauty Show in Long Beach, California. Prior to our first salon trade show, we assumed that all beauty professionals would have beautiful, symmetrical eyebrows. They did not.

Instead, what we found was that many professionals and students did not possess the knowledge base needed to perform successful eyebrow enhancement. The professionals shared their uncertainty and fears with us about performing eyebrow enhancement services for their clients. We found this to be true in cities all across the country and in countries throughout the world.

Realizing the need for a complete "how-to" resource on the subject of eyebrows, the company changed its focus from selling eyebrow enhancement products to educating students and beauty professionals on how to provide this service to clients.

There is no prerequisite knowledge needed for this course of study. It is a comprehensive resource that begins with the basics of facial beauty and culminates with the execution of the perfect brow. Therefore, it is not just for the seasoned professional but also for the student of every beauty discipline.

Organization and Features of the Text

In the first five chapters, time-tested rules and theories regarding facial features are examined and discussed. Where differences of opinion exist, the options are analyzed and explained. This lays the foundation for the last eight chapters of the book.

Chapter 6 introduces and teaches the process of assessing the eyebrow to determine color, texture, and other characteristics that allow the professional to prepare the eyebrow for shaping and design.

Chapter 7 provides the all-important core of information, the rules of proper eyebrow placement. Building on that knowledge, Chapter 8 details corrective techniques that can be performed on the eyebrows to enhance the other features of the face. Chapters 9 and 10 focus on the different methods a professional can use to perform an eyebrow makeover.

Hair removal experts share their knowledge in Chapter 11 to provide the reader with the most current trends and techniques in each method. In Chapter 12, other specialty services related to eyebrow enhancement are examined such as permanent makeup. State-of-the-art information from experts in these specialty disciplines is also included in the text.

Case studies are provided in Chapter 13. This significant chapter synthesizes all of the information from previous chapters and puts it to practical use. The students of eyebrow enhancement will see and further learn from the utilization of the techniques as they witness the dramatic impact that a well-designed eyebrow can create.

The text is interspersed with quizzes, charts, professional tips, photographs, and drawings to assist the student and the beauty professional in the learning process.

The best use of this text is to read and study it in the order in which it is written. This is because each chapter builds on the knowledge of the previous chapters. Use the suggested tools for the maximum learning experience and step through each suggested task, resisting the temptation to skip to the later chapters.

Regardless of your prior experience, you are about to learn and develop new skills that have been mastered only by a select few in your field. You are poised to begin acquiring the much sought-after eyebrow enhancement techniques that will broaden your talents and deepen your overall knowledge of beauty refinement. Enjoy the process of becoming a Master Eyebrow Specialist.

To verify and validate mastery of eyebrow design principles, the reader can take the Master Eyebrow Specialist test, which was produced and compiled by the experts at Adriel, Inc. Upon receiving a score of 90 percent or better, each candidate will receive his or her Master Eyebrow Design Specialist certification from Adriel, Inc. The test can be accessed at www.perfectbrow.com.

The following professionals have graciously provided their expertise on the subject of hair removal and other eyebrow related services for Chapters 11 and 12.

Tweezing Expert:
Rhonda G. Thomson
Face & Body Essence Skin Care
Fort Wayne, Indiana

Waxing Expert:
Lori Nestore
Eva's Esthetics
Oakland, California
www.thewaxqueen.com

Sugaring Expert:
Lina Kennedy
Alexandria Professional Body Sugaring
Welland, Ontario, Canada
www.alexandriasugaring.com

Threading Expert:
Shobha Tummala
Just Shobha Salon
Eyes of the World, Inc.
New York, New York
www.shobhathreading.com

Laser Expert:
Omeed Memar, M.D., Ph.D.
Academic Dermatology & Skin Cancer Institute
Chicago, Illinois
www.adsci.com

Permanent Makeup Expert:
Rose Marie Beauchemin
The Beau Institute of Permanent &
    Corrective Cosmetics
Mt. Laurel, New Jersey
www.beauinstitute.com

Tinting Expert:
Karen Wallace
Grace College of Cosmetology
Middleburg Heights, Ohio

Special thanks to:

Linda Rice, Karen Wallace, and all the students and professionals at Grace College of Cosmetology for their assistance with the photo shoot.

Kathleen Weiss for her expertise in editing the book.

Karen Wallace whose expertise is unbounded and who is among the best educators.

Judy Roberts and Eileen Clawson of Milady for their expertise, professionalism, and support throughout this project.

Larry Hamill for sharing his amazing abilities in photography, and for his patience and wonderful sense of humor during the photo shoot.

Heather Stankewicz for sharing her talents in makeup artistry.

And Anne and John Everson for their sound advice.

The author and editors at Milady recognize with respect and gratitude the following educators and professionals who have played a part in the development of this book:

Linzi Biesinger
Altoona Beauty School
Altoona, Pennsylvania

Stacy Heatherly
Image Enhancers
Papillion, Nebraska

Ruby Howard
Pinecrest High School
Cameron, North Carolina

Sharon MacGregor
Bloomingburg, New York

Katherine Phelps
Moore Norman Technology Center
Norman, Oklahoma

Martha Phillips
Ford Beauty Academy
Lowellville, Ohio

Rebecca Moran
Cumberland, Maine

Helen Bickmore
Jean Paul Spa
Albany, New York

Vickie Landess
BJ Salons Inc.
Springfield, Illinois

Carol McAllister
Bishop State Community College
Mobile, Alabama

Judith Holmes
Maricopa Beauty College
Avondale, Arizona

Deborah Beatty
Columbus Technical College
Columbus, Alabama

Victoria Bush is a licensed esthetician, color specialist, and makeup artist. She is a member of the Aesthetics' International Association (AIA). Her career in makeup artistry began in the early 1980s when she worked as a makeup artist for some of the large retail cosmetic companies. She traveled to various major cities, including New York and Los Angeles, attending seminars and training in makeup artistry.

Ms. Bush graduated summa cum laude from Georgia State University with a degree in Finance and a minor concentration in English and Literature.

Her varied and extensive background includes working as an analyst for two large corporations, selling both commercial and residential real estate, performing public and media relations duties for several political candidates, acting as editor for a local political newspaper, and writing news articles and press releases for both corporate and political entities.

It was during the early 1990s when Ms. Bush began to focus on one of the more prominent features of her appearance, the eyebrows. She spent countless dollars and hours trying to find a beauty specialist who could tame and beautify her thick, full eyebrows. She went to salons, spas, electrologists, and other makeup artists, but no one could give her the beautiful, symmetrical eyebrows she had always wanted.

She began an intense research program to learn everything about the elusive "perfect brow." In 1998, she and her husband created a system that would allow her to have beautiful eyebrows everyday. Realizing its market potential, she founded Adriel, Inc., and began marketing her Brow Perfection eyebrow enhancement products.

On learning about Brow Perfection products, Tweezerman Corporation extended an invitation to Adriel, Inc. to demonstrate and sell Brow Perfection products at the prestigious International Beauty Show (IBS) in Long Beach, California. The show was a complete success and Adriel, Inc. began selling and distributing its professional products through all of the major trade shows, including the IBS in New York and the BBSI in Las Vegas.

During that time, Victoria Bush performed thousands and thousands of "eyebrow designs" and makeovers. She conducted seminars at trade shows, salon locations, and private distributorships. She wrote articles for major industry magazines such as *Dermascope* and *Beauty Beat* on the subject of eyebrow enhancement. It was this practical, hands-on experience that taught her the many principles and original ideas that she shares in her book.

While traveling across the country, she learned firsthand that many beauty professionals were afraid to perform eyebrow enhancement work because they did not understand some of the basic beauty and eyebrow enhancement principles. She consistently received (and still receives) letters and e-mails from beauty schools and beauty professionals around the world asking her to come and teach them all about eyebrows.

Realizing the difficulty involved with personally teaching each and every professional, she set to work to write the definitive book on eyebrow enhancement. The result of her years of study, research, and hands-on experience is this complete and authoritative book, *How to Create the Perfect Eyebrow*.

Chapter 1

THE ART AND SCIENCE OF CREATING BEAUTIFUL, SYMMETRICAL EYEBROWS

Learning Objectives

After reading this chapter, you should be able to:

1. Describe the benefits of a well-shaped eyebrow.

2. Define the term "eyebrow design," and describe the benefit of separating design and hair removal services.

3. Identify the tools needed for successful eyebrow enhancement.

4. Explain the sanitary considerations for each tool.

Altering the Eyebrow: A Rite of Passage

It has been said that the most beautiful eyebrows are the most natural ones, the unaltered eyebrows that make every woman look unique, young, and beautiful (Figure 1–1).

Bobbi Brown, in her book *Bobbi Brown Beauty*, agrees. "You are born with a brow shape that works naturally with your eyes and face. Your brow's own natural line should be your guide." Not all experts agree, however. Nancy Parker, in her book *Beautiful Brows*, believes just the opposite. "No, your brow shape doesn't have to follow your natural brow line (that's like saying your hairstyle has to follow the natural flow of your hair)."

What the experts can agree on is that most women have somehow altered their original eyebrows either by tweezing, waxing, or electrolysis. This has lead to a large percentage of women having an asymmetrical or ill-designed eyebrow (Figure 1–2).

In our society and in other cultures, tweezing or altering one's eyebrows is a rite of passage into womanhood, much like wearing makeup for the first time or having one's ears pierced. The fact that women do and will continue to modify their eyebrows, coupled with their lack of expertise in doing so, creates a need for beauty professionals to study and learn the art and science of creating beautiful, symmetrical eyebrows.

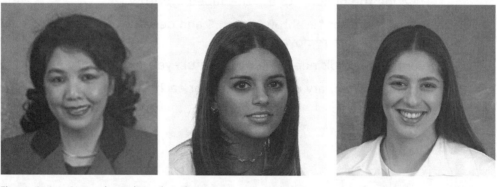

Figure 1–1.   Natural, unaltered eyebrows

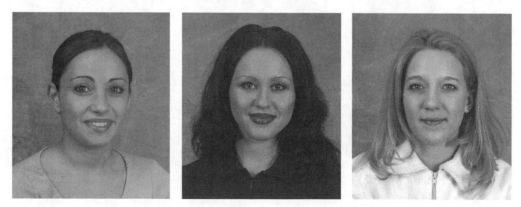

Figure 1–2.   Altered, asymmetrical eyebrows

Servicing All Nationalities and All Ages

As you study and learn the correct way to enhance and shape eyebrows, you will accumulate knowledge that is pertinent to all women's eyebrows, regardless of race, color, or age (Figure 1–3). While certain groups do possess similar eyebrow characteristics, it is not easy to categorize them because the pattern of similarities is inconsistent. The important concept is that the techniques for resolving eyebrow problems are the same, regardless of a person's nationality or age.

Ethnic and age differences do, however, affect methodology with respect to other disciplines in the fields of cosmetology and esthetics. For example, the methods, products, and techniques used on a white woman's hair can be significantly different from those used on an African American woman's hair. Because of this, you must study the many different types of hair in order to effectively provide hair services to any patron who comes into the salon.

Possessing the universally applicable knowledge of eyebrow enhancement allows you the opportunity to serve all clients, including people who have medical issues such as cancer, alopecia, or hair loss. Patients undergoing chemotherapy or radiation therapies often lose eyebrow hair in addition to hair on other parts of the body. Professionals who work with medical patients can provide them with an improved appearance by recreating their eyebrows as part of their overall medical therapy. This is what the volunteer professionals do who are involved with the Look Good, Feel Better program. This program, created out of an alliance between the American Cancer Society and volunteers from the beauty industry, assists patients with wigs, makeup, and other enhancements while they are undergoing treatments.

Whether you are recreating an eyebrow for a medical patient or repairing an overtweezed eyebrow, an eyebrow is an eyebrow is an eyebrow. Once you master this body of knowledge, you can perform this service on any person who comes to you, regardless of nationality, age, or health condition.

Losing Your Fear, Gaining Confidence

One of the most exciting parts of a beauty professional's work is solving problems for your clients. Whether a solution is found that provides a new haircolor, healthier skin, or a mended nail, helping each client brings great rewards for all parties involved.

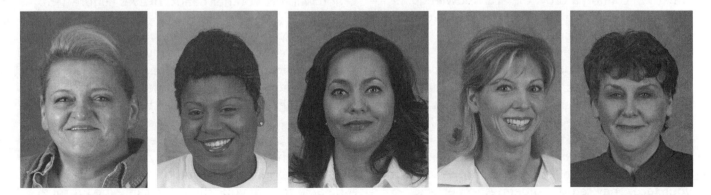

Figure 1–3.   Women of different ages and nationalities

When a client comes to you and you are unsure of how to approach her problem, fear and despair set in. Many beauty professionals cringe in fear when a client asks them to shape and enhance their eyebrows. The result of this debilitating fear is an ill-shaped, asymmetrical eyebrow, and a dissatisfied client who will not return to your salon.

This leads to the distinct purpose and objective of this book, which is to remove all fear and uncertainty and replace it with complete confidence gained only from knowledge and understanding. With your new confidence, you will expertly design a suitable and beautiful eyebrow for each client. This will allow for secure and confident hair removal each time the client comes to your salon or spa. Once you know how to enhance and perfect any pair of eyebrows, regardless of the abuse or neglect they have undergone, you will welcome every client to your chair.

Becoming a Brow Expert by Focusing on Eyebrow Design

As you study the techniques in this book and consistently practice them, you will be well on your way to becoming a brow expert. Knowledge, practice, and confidence are what differentiate the expert from the untrained professional.

There is plenty of room for more experts on the subject of eyebrows. But present experts in the business of beauty are consistent when it comes to the importance of eyebrows in the overall design and enhancement of facial beauty. From Rex, in the book *Making Up by Rex*, he says, "Balance is the key attribute well-shaped eyebrows can give your face. They're our guidelines to perfect makeup placement and as such you must make

sure their shape is right before you begin any other shaping or corrections. The length and arch of your brow will help you determine your base-shading technique, subtly influence the way your nose is perceived, and affect the placement of your eye makeup."

From Charlotte Tilbury, London makeup artist for a 2003 Prada fashion show, "Eyebrows are the pillars of the face. They broadcast a powerful message to the world about who you are."

From Bobbi Brown, in her book *Bobbi Brown Beauty*, ". . . a well-groomed, well-defined brow can be extremely flattering and add considerable strength to a woman's eyes. It can open up her face so that she actually needs less makeup. A well-shaped brow can also help lift deep-set eyes or maximize small eyes. There are even instances where a lifted, well-manicured brow has had the same effect as a surgical eyelift."

And from *Oprah Magazine*, in a recent article and photo layout featuring Anastasia Soare, "Eyebrows that are too thick, too thin, not long enough, or unruly can call so much attention to themselves that other prettier features go unnoticed."

If a woman's eyebrows are ill-shaped or asymmetrical, all of the attention will focus on her unattractive eyebrows (Figure 1–4). If a woman's eyebrows are symmetrical and well-groomed, all of the attention will focus on her beautiful eyes (Figure 1–5).

In order to progress from a student to an expert in eyebrow enhancement, you must separate "eyebrow design" from the hair removal service. "Eyebrow design" is the process of choosing and applying an ideal brow shape based on the client's features, and placing it in a location that enhances the client's appearance. If "eyebrow design" is performed efficiently, it need only be done one time during the initial consultation. Thereafter, you will be able to give your client the same, beautiful eyebrow at each subsequent appointment.

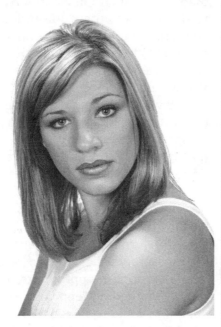

Figure 1–4.　The focus is on the unattractive eyebrows.

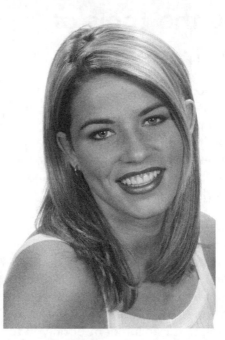

Figure 1–5.　The focus is on her beautiful eyes.

Your client will finally get the eyebrows she has always dreamed of, rather than holding her breath to "see what she'll get this time." Before long, word about your unique expertise will travel to the friends and relatives of your clients. They will quickly come to understand the difference between a "wax job" and an "eyebrow design" service, and will gladly pay the one-time consultation fee for your expertise.

Let's begin the journey as a student of eyebrow enhancement with an introduction to the tools needed to perform your work. The Resource Directory at the end of this book will guide you in locating the tools you wish to purchase.

HOW TO MAKE EYEBROW DESIGN WORK IN YOUR SALON

Create a separate fee for the "eyebrow design" service, which includes consulting with the client, choosing the best shape, applying corrective techniques, and maintaining the client's records. This fee should range from $20 and higher. Make sure the client understands that she will be charged the "eyebrow design" fee only one time. At each subsequent visit, the client will only pay the standard eyebrow hair removal fee.

Acquiring the Tools of the Brow Trade

As with any profession, it is necessary to have the right tools to provide the optimal service to your clients. Before the introduction of each eyebrow enhancement tool, it is necessary to become familiar with the agencies that provide the sanitary and safety regulations under which each professional and salon must work.

Each state's Board of Cosmetology deals with sanitary rules for salons and equipment, as well as licensing for salons and professionals. Their primary goal is to have the highest degree of public safety for all individuals in a salon setting. Because each state has different rules and regulations regarding sanitation in the salon, it is incumbent upon you to contact your state Board of Cosmetology to receive a copy of your state's Salon Sanitation Rules and Regulations.

In addition, each state has its own Occupational Safety and Health Administration (OSHA) office. OSHA's focus is broad and includes protecting the safety of workers and patrons in all professions. OSHA has specific jurisdiction in the case of blood spills with respect to proper disinfecting and disposal of implements and/or equipment that comes in contact with bloodborne pathogens.

To locate your state Board of Cosmetology and your state's local OSHA office, refer to a textbook entitled *Safety and Health in the Salon* written by Dennis Nelson. This book outlines the proper safety procedures that should be followed by a beauty professional when performing eyebrow enhancements and other services.

The following are some general guidelines provided by Mr. Nelson with regard to the serious issue of cross-contamination: "Cosmetologists or estheticians need all of the equipment and procedures to decontaminate implements and machines used for facial and makeup services. Important infection control procedures include hand washing and sanitation, use of personal protective equipment (PPE) like gloves and safety glasses, and proper disinfecting of all implements and surfaces. You should never remove products from their containers with your fingers. Always use a clean spatula or new/clean applicator. Use only sanitized brushes and implements and a shaker-type container for loose powders. Pour all lotions from bottle containers. Use an antiseptic on tweezed areas of the eyebrow to avoid infection. Discard all disposable supplies and materials. Close and clean product containers and put them in their proper places. Return unused cosmetics and other items to the dispensary. Place used towels, coverlets, and head coverings in appropriate containers until they can be laundered. Keep your work area clean, neat, and well organized. Wash and sanitize your hands before each service, or after touching any object unrelated to the procedure."

As you become acquainted with and follow these regulations, you will be able to provide your clients with the services they desire in a clean and safe environment. For both the client and the professional, it is of the highest importance to follow sanitary and safety procedures with respect to each of the tools.

Tools

The **eyebrow brush/comb** (Figure 1–6) is used throughout the eyebrow enhancement process. It is used for combing the brow hairs while trimming them, for manipulating the eyebrow while assessing the characteristics of the eyebrow, and during hair removal to separate the hairs to be removed from the hairs that are to remain.

Sanitary Considerations: It is optimal to use a disposable eyebrow brush for each client. You may choose to give the client the eyebrow brush used only on them. If the eyebrow brush is to be reused, it should be washed in hot, soapy water, then disinfected in a solution for the appropriate length of time.

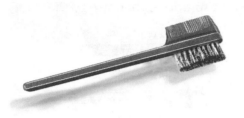

Figure 1–6. Eyebrow brush/comb

The *ruler* or *measuring device* (Figure 1–7) is used to assist beauty professionals in judging the eye set, the beginning and ending points of the eyebrow, and other valuable considerations. It should be no more than six inches long so it is easy to manipulate. It should be completely flat for pinpoint accuracy. Therefore, do not use objects like an orangewood stick or a pencil for measuring.

Sanitary Considerations: If the measuring device does not touch the client's skin, it is not necessary to sanitize it after each customer use. However, spraying the measuring device with alcohol will protect against bacterial growth. If the measuring device does touch the client's skin, immerse it in a disinfectant solution.

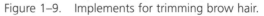

Figure 1–7. Ruler

Tweezers (Figure 1–8) can be used for the primary method of hair removal or as a secondary method when removing hairs left behind after performing a different method of hair removal. It is essential to have at least one high-quality pair of tweezers. They do not have to be expensive, but they need to be effective. If you have a pair that doesn't grasp the hair each time, it is time to invest in a new pair.

Sanitary Considerations: Tweezers must be sanitized or sterilized after each client. If blood is present, follow your state's Board of Cosmetology guidelines for sanitizing implements that have come into contact with blood.

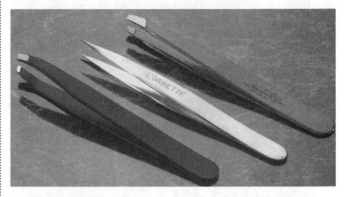

Figure 1–8. Tweezers

As with tweezers, it is critical to have good quality *scissors* or *nippers* (Figure 1–9) for trimming brow hairs. Small scissors are often used for this purpose. You can also use cuticle nippers, which are more stable because the built-in, springy resistance provides a small but constant pressure in your hand during the trimming process. The sanitary considerations are the same as those for tweezers.

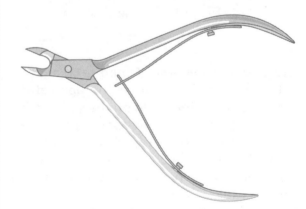

Figure 1–9. Implements for trimming brow hair.

Eyebrow powders (Figure 1–10) are used for filling in the bare or sparse areas of the eyebrow to create symmetry and enhance the existing shape. They can also be used to temporarily change the color of the eyebrows as they come in a variety of colors. Your basic palette of colors should include dark brown, medium brown, light brown, taupe, medium gray, light gray, yellow, light auburn, and dark auburn. Eyebrow powders are flat, not frosted. A frosted or shimmering eyebrow would not look natural. The matte finish of the brow powder allows it to stay on longer.

Sanitary Considerations: For each client, remove a small amount of powder of each color needed with a disposable spatula into a clean dish or palette. Dipping into a compact after touching the client's skin is not a sanitary practice, and will transfer bacteria to and from the compact to the skin of each client.

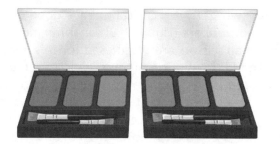

Figure 1–10.   Eyebrow powders in an array of colors and values

Eyebrow powder applicators (Figure 1–11) are either soft or stiff. The brush on the soft applicator has rounded bristles. The brush on the stiff applicator has angled bristles. The soft applicator will deposit more powder to the area, while the stiff applicator will deposit a lighter amount of powder in a more limited area. Also, some applicators have long handles while others have shorter handles. The choice of handle length is based on cost and preference.

Sanitary Considerations: Disposable applicators are optimal. If you choose to reuse the applicator brush, then it must be washed in warm,

soapy water, then sanitized in a disinfectant solution. The disinfectant solution must be thoroughly rinsed from the brush because disinfectant solution is harmful to the skin.

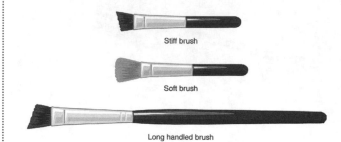
Stiff brush

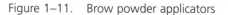
Soft brush

Long handled brush

Figure 1–11.   Brow powder applicators

A *thin tipped artist's brush* (Figure 1–12) can also be used to apply eyebrow powder. Dip the brush into a container of clean water, then dab the brush into a small amount of brow powder that has been removed from the compact. You can apply the wet powder in hair-like strokes for a natural look.

Sanitary Considerations: A disposable brush is optimal. If you choose to reuse the brush, sanitize it properly according to your state's sanitary regulations.

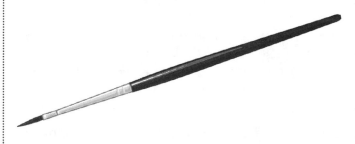

Figure 1–12.   Brush applicator for use with wet eyebrow powder

Eyebrow pencils (Figure 1–13) are the most common choice for fill-in. The benefits of using pencil over powder are that the fill-in can be done more quickly and that an eyebrow pencil is more easily portable than a compact of powder, a spatula, and a palette.

Sanitary Considerations: Sharpen the eyebrow pencil thoroughly between clients so as not to transfer bacteria from one client to the next. Optimally, one should break off the tip of the pencil after each client before sharpening it. The sharpener must also be sanitized after each client. Replace the pencil cap when it is not in use to prevent bacteria from getting into the pencil.

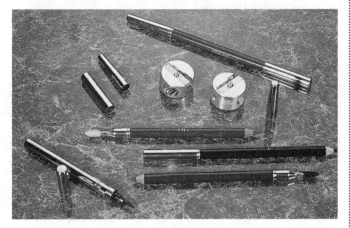

Figure 1–13. Eyebrow pencils in a variety of colors

Setting the eyebrow with a *brow gel* or *cream* (Figure 1–14) after applying powder or pencil is an essential step in the eyebrow enhancement process. This is done to ensure that the brow hairs do not move out of place and accidentally change the shape of a well-designed eyebrow. Brow setting gels come in a variety of forms. Some come in a mascara-like tube with a wand. Others are in the form of a cream that must be applied with an eyebrow brush.

Sanitary Considerations: If you use the brow setting gel in a tube with a wand, use two or more disposable wands for each client. You must use one disposable wand for each eyebrow since you should not reenter the tube with a wand that has touched the client's skin. If you use the cream in a separate tube with an eyebrow brush/comb, be sure to dispose of the brush after each use or give it to the client. If you wish

to reuse the eyebrow brush, immerse it in a disinfectant solution and thoroughly rinse it after the specified time of immersion.

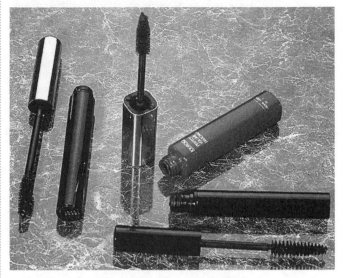

Figure 1–14. Brow setting products

Templates (Figure 1–15) serve as a guide when the client's eyebrows require fill-in. The template is most beneficial to the client who needs to perform fill-in every day. The eyebrow shape on the template must be chosen based on systematic measuring as outlined in the chapters. Use templates from a company that provides a wide array of choices in thickness and length, and that gives you the actual length measurements and thickness specifications.

Sanitary Considerations: It is optimal to use one template per customer. If this is not possible, the templates must be disinfected with alcohol.

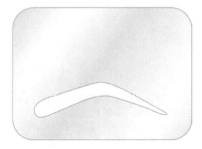

Figure 1–15. Plastic templates with the eyebrow shape "punched out"

Brow perfecting strips (Figure 1–16) are like templates in that they are imbedded with an eyebrow shape that provides a guideline for the "eyebrow design" and hair removal processes. The difference is that the strips temporarily adhere to the skin or to the brow, whereas the templates must be held in place.

Sanitary Considerations: Always use one pair of strips per customer and dispose of them after each use.

In addition to these eleven tools used in the eyebrow design process, you may wish to acquire different hair removal equipment and implements. Whichever equipment and/or methods you choose for hair removal purposes, you must know how to use each item and how to properly sanitize it for the highest customer satisfaction and safety.

We now turn our attention to assessing the facial features and the eyebrows. After mastering these assessments, we will begin to work with your new eyebrow enhancement toolbox.

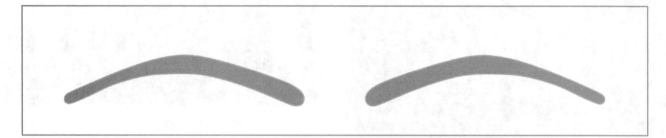

Figure 1–16. Brow perfecting strips

REFERENCES

Monroe, V. (2003, February). The eyebrow experiment. *The Oprah Magazine*, 174–179.

Brown, B., & Iverson, A. (1997). *Bobbi Brown beauty: The ultimate beauty resource.* New York: HarperStyle.

Jewell, D. L. (1986). *Making up by Rex: Beauty for every age, every woman.* New York: Clarkson Potter/Publishers.

Lamont, E. (2003, October). High brow. Can changing your eyebrows change your face—and the way the world perceives you? *Vogue, 388,* 413.

Nelson, D. (2001). *Safety and health in the salon: Facilitator's guide.* Clifton Park, NY: Delmar Learning.

Parker, N., & Kalish, N. (2000). *Beautiful brows: The ultimate guide to styling, shaping, and maintaining your eyebrows.* New York: Three Rivers Press.

Chapter 2

THE STUDY OF THE FACIAL ZONES

Learning Objectives

After reading this chapter, you should be able to:

1. Identify and define the three facial zones.

2. List the advantages of understanding how to study a client's facial zones.

3. Define symmetry and beauty in relation to symmetry.

4. Describe the midpoint of the face and how it is used.

Tools you will need:

- a ruler
- a pencil for drawing and plotting

The face can be divided into zones in order to help you clearly identify areas that are proportionally wide or long. Studying and measuring to find the client's facial zones will provide you with two benefits.

1. You will be able to see which zones are long and which are wide in order to perform corrective techniques in hair styling and with makeup.
2. You will be able to more clearly identify the face shape of the client.

Before we begin the study of the facial zones, it is necessary to discuss the importance of symmetry with respect to the overall appearance of the face.

Symmetry of the Face

Symmetry is defined as "similarity of form or arrangement on either side of a dividing line . . . a correspondence of opposite parts in size, shape, and position." Beauty is defined as "excellence of form as a result of such correspondence." Facial symmetry occurs or is achieved when the size, shape, and position of features is even on both sides of the face.

The significant conclusion is that the more symmetry you can create, the more perceived beauty exists. Features can be made to look more symmetrical through the proper and intelligent use of cosmetics, not the least of which occurs in eyebrow enhancement.

For each face you study and desire to improve, imagine a line running directly down the middle. We will refer to this line as the midpoint of the face (Figure 2–1). When you are studying the features of a client's face, note those features that are symmetrical and those that are not. For example, are the eyes the same size, shape, and distance apart from the midpoint? Are the lips the same shape, length, and thickness on both sides? Do both eyebrows have the same thickness, shape, and height above the eyes? This information will be useful when performing corrective techniques to eyebrow shaping and to all cosmetic applications.

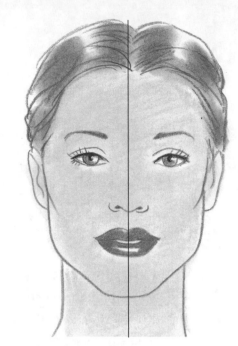

Figure 2–1.   Imaginary line shows the midpoint of the face

While no one's facial features are perfectly symmetrical, using makeup to give the illusion of symmetry will dramatically improve a person's overall appearance. As a beauty professional, one of your main goals is to create facial symmetry.

Marvin Westmore, founder of The Westmore Academy of Cosmetic Arts in Burbank, California, emphasizes the importance of balance and symmetry in his collection of articles, entitled, "The ABC of Eyebrow Design." Westmore writes, "The eyebrows are the most visible facial feature where imbalance and asymmetry is obvious. Since we draw attention to the eyebrows repeatedly by using them to add emphasis to our words or to express our feelings silently, it is important that the brows be as realistically symmetrical as possible, providing maximum facial beauty and non-verbal communication capabilities."

Anastasia Soare, Beverly Hills salon owner and eyebrow stylist to some of the world's most famous faces, also emphasizes the importance of eyebrows with respect to facial symmetry. "My goal is to make the eyebrows beautifully symmetrical be-cause even when features are asymmetrical—as they most often are—well-shaped brows will bring a kind of harmony to the face."

The Three Facial Zones

The face is divided lengthwise (from top to bot-tom) into three zones (Figure 2–2). The upper zone is measured from the hairline to just below the eyebrow at its beginning point. The middle zone is measured from that point at the eyebrows to the base of the nose. The lower zone is measured from the base of the nose to the bottom of the chin.

Take note of the features that are in each zone. The upper zone consists of the forehead and the eyebrows. The middle zone contains the eyes and the nose. The lower zone contains the lips and

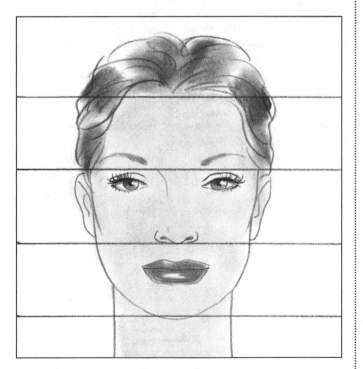

Figure 2–2.   The three facial zones

chin. All three zones are impacted by and have an impact on the hairstyle that is worn by the person.

This information is particularly useful as you begin to study the different facial features in Chapter 5, and understand the impact of making cosmetic changes to these features in Chapter 8.

Measuring the Facial Zones to Determine the Length and Width of the Face

To correctly measure the length and width of a client's face and determine her geometric face shape, you must make a two-dimensional (length and width) assessment. In other words, measure the face as if it has no depth, just as you would a picture in a magazine. Therefore, use a ruler and not a soft tape measure to make the assessments.

When measuring the facial zones, make three lengthwise (top to bottom) measurements and four width-wise (side to side) measurements. The meas-urements are based on the divisions of the face as pictured in Figure 2–2. To obtain measurements for the length of the face, measure the upper, middle, and lower zones vertically, as close to the midpoint of the face as possible. To obtain the four measure-ments needed for the width of the face, measure across the face (side to side) at the four different vertical points on the face.

1. The top of the forehead (the hairline)
2. At the underside of the eyebrow
3. At the base of the nose
4. At the chin

STEP-BY-STEP: Measuring the Facial Zones

STEP 1: Pull hair back completely away from the face. This is absolutely essential because the hairline must be measured accurately to determine the length of the face. It is also necessary to see the hairline in order to correctly determine the face shape.

STEP 2: With a ruler, measure the three facial zones vertically from top to bottom (Figures 2–3, 2–4, and 2–5). Measure as close to the middle of the face as possible and make a two-dimensional measurement. Record the information below.

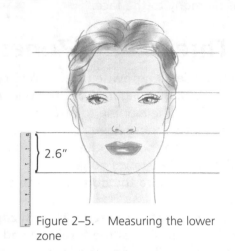

Figure 2–5.   Measuring the lower zone

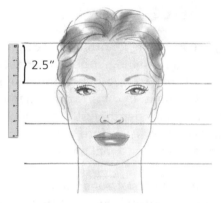

Figure 2–3.   Measuring the upper zone

Upper Zone (from hairline to eyebrow) _____

Middle Zone (from eyebrow to base of nose)_____

Lower Zone (from base of nose to chin) _____

Total Length of the Face (sum of upper, middle, and lower zones) _____

STEP 3: With a ruler, measure from side to side at the hairline (Figure 2–6), the eyebrow, the base of the nose, and the chin. Once again, this measurement is difficult because it must be done as though there is no depth to the

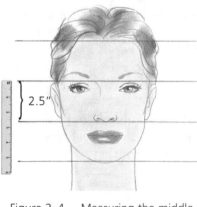

Figure 2–4.   Measuring the middle zone

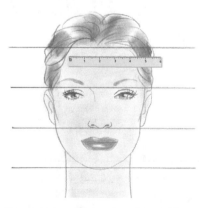

Figure 2–6.   Measuring the width at the hairline

face. Therefore, measure from side to side that which is visible to the eye. Ideally, you should have someone measure your facial zones just as you would do for your clients.

Record the width measurements here.

Hairline width _____

At eyebrow width_____

At base of nose width _____

At chin width _____

STEP 4: Make a rough drawing using the vertical measurements obtained in Step 2. Use Figure 2–7 to assist you in making the rough drawing. Begin at the center of the page, and using the ruler, vertically plot the points for the hairline, the eyebrow, the base of the nose, and the chin.

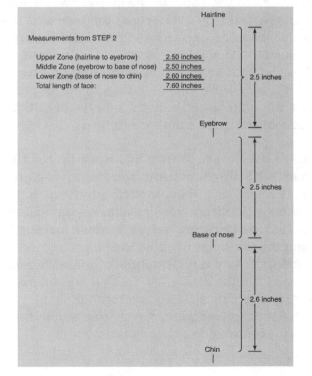

Figure 2–7.   Plotting the zones

STEP 5: On the rough drawing created in Step 4, use the four marks as the midpoint of the face. At each point, draw width-wise each of the four measurements obtained in Step 3 (see Figure 2–8). The first mark is for the hairline width, the second is for the "at eyebrow" width, and so on. Remember to make the halfway point of the measurement intersect at the midpoint of the face. For example, if the hairline width is four inches, draw two inches to the left of the top mark and two inches to the right of the top mark.

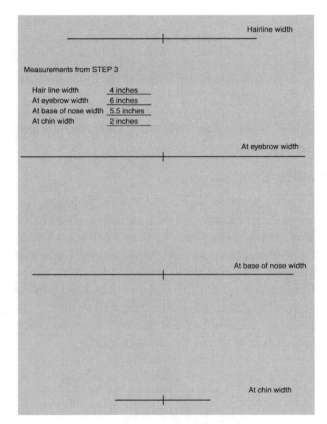

Figure 2–8.   Plotting the width measurements

STEP 6: On the rough drawing, create the frame of the face by connecting the lines with either curved or straight lines to copy the face (Figure 2–9).

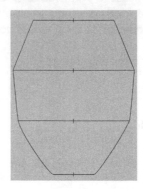

Figure 2–9.   Connect the lines to show the frame of the face

By performing these six steps, you will be able to see the length and width of a face, and more easily distinguish the geometric face shape.

Practice Exercise

In order to practice measuring the facial zones, choose a person and measure and record the following information. Then turn to Figure 2–10 and plot and draw that person's facial zones. Once that is complete, connect the outside points with either straight or curved lines to copy your subject's face. This exercise will train you to assess the zones and shape of a face without the use of a ruler by teaching you which parts of the face to study.

Corrective Techniques Based on Length and Width

While some beauty professionals perform corrective techniques based on the face shape assess-

ment, others prefer to use only length and width proportions for this purpose. Knowing the length and width of the zones of the face will allow you to understand which corrections can be made. Dutifully measuring and recording the information as outlined in the above steps will not be necessary after you become experienced at assessing your client's faces. However, it is a useful fallback procedure when presented with the unusual or difficult case that can occur from time to time.

One of the most renowned makeup artists of our time, Dick Smith, uses width and length measurements when performing corrective techniques. In a timeless article from *Vogue* magazine, dated October 1957, he discusses "simple, sensible makeup," using the principles of addition and subtraction. "Where the face is wide, subtract; where it's meager, add." In the article, Mr. Smith shares his expertise regarding shading and contouring techniques, as well as the hairstyle selections he uses to correct wide and long facial zones.

Measurements from Step 2:

Upper Zone (from hairline to eyebrow) _____
Middle Zone (from eyebrow to base of nose) _____
_____
Lower Zone (from base of nose to chin) _____
_____
Total Length of Face (add all zones together) _____
_____

Measurements from Step 3:

Hairline width _____
At eyebrow width _____
At base of nose width_____
At chin width_____

Hairline
|

Figure 2–10.   Practice sheet

Dick Smith has been a professional makeup artist and consultant for over 50 years. He was head of the New York NBC-TV Make-up Department from 1945 to 1959 and has applied makeup to some of the most famous Hollywood faces. His makeup work in movies includes A Christmas Carol, Miracle on 34th Street, Mrs. Miniver, The Godfather Part 2, The Stepford Wives, Marathon Man, The Deer Hunter, Prizzi's Honor, Poltergeist III, *and hundreds of other films and television programs. One of his students, Rick Baker, who himself is an Oscar-winning makeup artist, calls Dick Smith "the greatest makeup artist living." To learn more about Dick Smith, visit his Web site at http://www.dicksmithmake-up.com.*

Quiz—The Facial Zones and Symmetry

1. Facial symmetry equates to _____ perceived beauty.
   A. more
   B. no difference in
   C. less

2. To analyze the face to see where it is symmetrical, use the _____ .
   A. facial zone measurements
   B. geometric face shape determination
   C. imaginary line called the midpoint of the face

3. The lower zone measures from the _____ to the _____ .

4. The upper zone measures from the _____ to _____ .

5. The middle zone measures from the _____ to the _____ .

6. Why is it important to know the facial zone measurements?
   A. To assist in determining geometric face shape
   B. To assist in more effectively performing cosmetic corrections
   C. Neither a or b
   D. Both a and b

REFERENCES

Monroe, V. (2003, February). The eyebrow experiment. *The Oprah Magazine*, 174–179.

D'Angelo, J., Lees, M., Dean, P. S., Miller, E., Dietz, S., Zani, A., & Hinds, C. 2003. *Milady's standard comprehensive training for estheticians.* Clifton Park, NY: Delmar Learning.

Smith, D. (1957, October). How to find your own beauty: With face-searching facts from NBC TV's make-up chief. *Vogue*, 61–62,143.

Westmore, M. G. (1995). *The ABC of eyebrow design.* Carol Stream, IL: Allured Publishing Corporation.

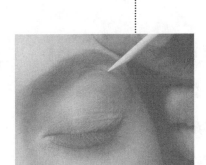

Chapter 3

THE STUDY OF THE GEOMETRIC FACE SHAPES

Learning Objectives

After reading this chapter, you should be able to:

1. List the four most commonly used face shapes.

2. List the four additional face shapes that are used by some beauty professionals.

3. Identify the one face shape that is considered to be the ideal geometric face shape.

4. Identify length and width characteristics for each of the eight face shapes.

5. Discuss appropriate corrective techniques for each face shape.

6. Look at photographs of real faces and determine the face shape.

Why Study the Different Face Shapes?

The traditional notion is that the oval face is the ideal geometric face shape when defining classic beauty. The oval face is considered to be the most well proportioned and perfectly balanced of all of the shapes.

Makeup theory and application, hair cutting and styling, plastic surgery, and all facial enhancement techniques have traditionally been taught with one objective in mind: to manipulate hair, makeup, skin, bone, and cartilage so that the face appears to be oval. In order for you to decide whether you will use the oval face shape as the benchmark of beauty in your work, you must learn and test the theory for yourself. Once you accomplish this, you can determine if its use actually assists you in performing your craft better than you otherwise would.

It is important to study and learn the different face shapes:

- to allow you to identify the face shape of a client.
- to allow you to see how it differs from the classic oval shape.
- to see more clearly the cosmetic changes you may wish to make.

What Are the Different Geometric Face Shapes and How Many Are There?

There are many different opinions as to the number and names of the different face shapes. Each textbook, magazine article, and beauty professional offers a different opinion. The different face shape theories fall into three categories.

1. No face shapes
2. Four basic face shapes
3. Seven or eight face shapes

No Face Shapes

There are some beauty professionals who ascribe to the belief that specific face shapes cannot be categorized. One or more of the following reasons may account for this opinion.

1. They find it too difficult to study, learn, and apply face shape theory.
2. They make the assessment and correction all in one step. In other words, they see the same things but prefer not to assess and categorize a face before making the corrections. This type of beauty professional usually makes the same corrections as the person who works with face shape theory, but does so more from instinct than from learned information.
3. They do not believe the traditional notion that the oval face is the epitome of all beauty. They see each face as a blank canvas, to be manipu-

---

SPECIAL NOTE:

It is recommended that you allow clients to help determine which features they would like to enhance. Rather than you making a judgment of their "undesirable" features, allow them to explain what characteristics of their appearance they dislike and would like to change.

lated with makeup and hairstyle to achieve a unique, personal look.

The Four Basic Face Shapes: Oval, Long, Square, and Round

Many beauty professionals utilize the four basic face shapes. Using four face shapes instead of more simplifies the process, making it easier to learn and utilize. All classifications of face shape—either four, seven, or eight—include the basic four of oval, long, square, and round.

The following is a detailed description of each of the face shapes, beginning with the four basic face shapes. Each face shape description is followed by a simplified list of corrective techniques that are often performed to make that particular face shape appear more oval.

The Oval Face Shape (Figure 3–1). This shape resembles an egg, with the smallest width of the egg in the lower zone. The hairline is rounded and is wider than the lower zone. The middle zone is the widest.

Corrective Techniques for the Oval Face Shape: None.

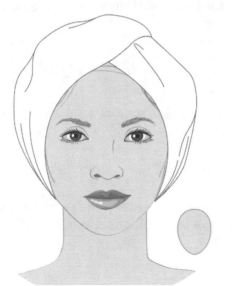

Figure 3–1.   The oval-shaped face

The Long Face Shape (Figure 3–2). This face shape is sometimes referred to as "oblong." All three zones have the same approximate width. The hairline is horizontal and goes from temple to temple. This face shape always has a length greater than its width.

Corrective Techniques for the Long Face Shape: Use techniques to give the illusion that a specific zone is either wider or shorter than it actually is. Either approach will make a zone look "less long."

For example, if the upper zone is longer than the other zones on a long face, you may choose to design an eyebrow shape with an arch at the outer part of the brow. You may also choose to apply eye makeup that extends beyond the outer corner of the eye. Either one of these corrections will make the upper zone appear wider, and hence, "less long."

You can create the illusion of shortening the upper zone by designing an eyebrow shape with very little arch height. This approach will also make the upper zone appear "less long."

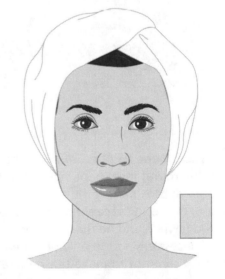

Figure 3–2.   The long- or oblong-shaped face

The Square Face Shape (Figure 3–3). Characterized by a squared jawline and hairline, this face shape is similar to the long face shape. The difference is the square-shaped face has a length and width that are approximately equal.

Corrective Techniques for the Square Face Shape: To make a square-shaped face appear more oval, apply makeup to the upper zone and the lower zone to round and narrow those areas. Also, slightly elongating one or more of the zones will make it appear more oval.

Using shading techniques, applying makeup in specific ways to the eyes and lips, and performing thoughtful eyebrow design techniques are ways makeup can be used to give the illusion of making these changes.

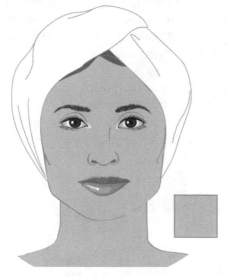

Figure 3–3.   The square-shaped face

The Round Face Shape (Figure 3–4). Like the square face shape, the round face shape has a length and width that are approximately the same. Unlike the square shape, the round face shape is characterized by a rounded jawline and hairline. A round face shape is not necessarily found only on a heavier set person, so take care not to make this generalization.

Corrective Techniques for the Round Face Shape: The corrections are similar to those for a square face shape, and include creating the illusion of lengthening the face and narrowing the upper

and lower zones. Use the makeup techniques listed for the square face shape.

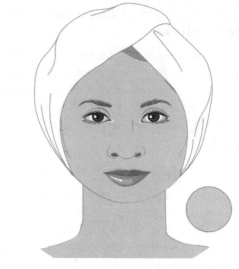

Figure 3–4.   The round-shaped face

Quiz–The Four Basic Face Shapes

1. Which face shape always has a length greater than its width?
   A. square
   B. round
   C. long
   D. oval

2. This shape is characterized with a middle zone having the widest measurement.
   A. square
   B. round
   C, long
   D. oval

3. There are no corrective techniques indicated with this face shape.
   A. square
   B. round
   C. long
   D. oval

4. This face shape has a squared jawline, and all three facial zones have approximately the same length and width.
   A. square
   B. round
   C. long
   D. oval

Seven or Eight Face Shapes

With a firm understanding of the four basic face shapes, it is easy to add three or four more to complete the study. Each textbook generally contains seven or eight face shapes, sometimes with different names and variations.

Seven Face Shapes = The Basic Four

1. oval
2. long
3. square
4. round

+ Three More

5. heart or inverted triangle
6. diamond
7. pear or triangle

Eight Face Shapes = The Basic Four

1. oval
2. long
3. square
4. round

+ Four More

5. heart or inverted triangle
6. diamond
7. pear or triangle
8. hexagon

The Heart or Inverted Triangle Face Shape (Figures 3–5 and 3–6). The upper zone is the widest, the middle zone is less wide than the upper zone, and the lower zone is the narrowest. The lower zone at the chin is more pointed than flat or round. The hairline is horizontal and wide from temple to temple. This wide hairline causes the face to take on the inverted triangle shape as opposed to the diamond or oval shape. The length of the zones is often approximately the same.

The inverted triangle face shape becomes a heart shape when the hairline has a widow's peak (Figure 3–5) instead of horizontal hairline (Figure 3–6).

Corrective Techniques for the Heart or Inverted Triangle Face Shape: Make the upper zone appear narrower and more rounded to resemble that of an oval. This can be done by shading, altering the hairstyle, changing arch placement to the eyebrows, or any other method that has a narrowing effect in the upper zone.

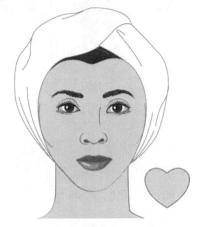

Figure 3–5.   The heart-shaped face

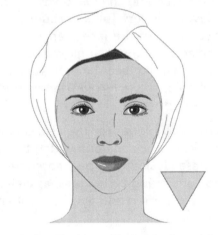

Figure 3–6.   The inverted triangle-shaped face

The Diamond-Shaped Face (Figure 3–7). Characterized by a hairline and a chin that are equally narrow, this shape has a middle zone that is clearly the widest of the three zones.

Corrective Techniques for the Diamond Face Shape: Make corrections to create the illusion of widening the upper and lower zones to resemble an oval. This can be done by contouring around the temples and the jawline, shading the middle zone (cheek), changing the arch location of the eyebrow, and using other corrective methods.

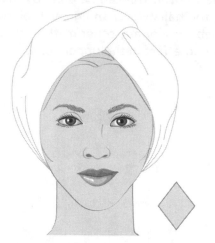

Figure 3–7.   The diamond-shaped face

The Pear-Shaped Face (Figure 3–8). This is the widest at the chin and the narrowest at the hairline. The jawline is very full and rounded. This is the least common of the face shapes and is sometimes referred to as the triangle-shaped face. (Note that a triangle face shape has the point at the top, whereas the inverted triangle has the point at the bottom.)

Corrective Techniques for the Pear-Shaped Face: Narrow the lower zone and widen the upper zone. These illusions can be created with shading and contouring techniques, as well as with makeup application and eyebrow enhancement techniques.

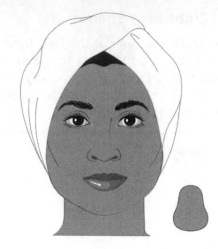

Figure 3–8.   The pear-shaped face

The Hexagonal Face Shape (Figure 3–9). This face shape is quite similar to the oval-shaped face except that it is angular where the oval is more rounded. Angles exist at the temples and the jawline, and the cheekbone area as well. This face shape appears to have six straight sides with the hairline horizontally flat. The hairline does not go from temple to temple, making it less wide than the middle zone, which is the widest.

Corrective Techniques for the Hexagonal Face Shape: Since this shape is similar to an oval face shape, only a softening of the angles may be desired. This can be successfully accomplished by shading the angled areas.

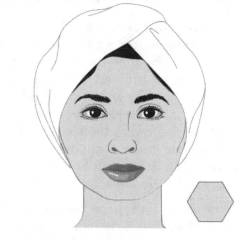

Figure 3–9.   The hexagon-shaped face

Face Shape Chart

Figure 3–10 is a chart of the different face shapes and is a useful tool when working to identify a client's face shape.

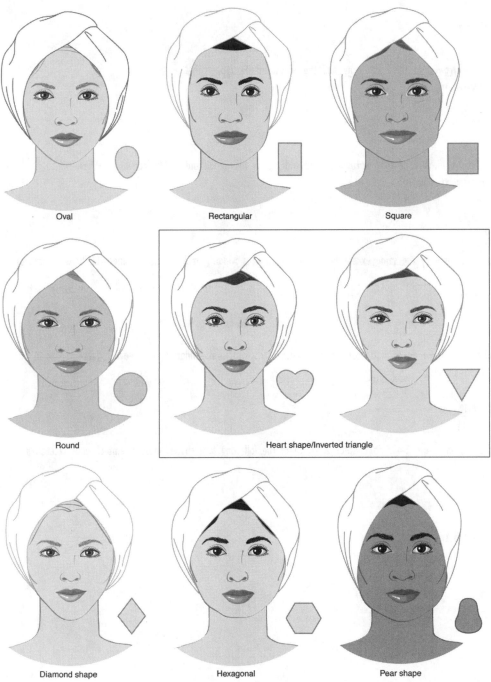

Figure 3–10.   Face shape chart—Eight geometric face shapes

Quiz—The Four Additional Face Shapes

1. This face shape is characterized by a pointed hairline and chin, and has a middle zone that is wider than the other zones.
   - A. heart or inverted triangle
   - B. diamond
   - C. pear or triangle
   - D. hexagon

2. Which shape is the narrowest in the lower zone and the widest in the upper zone?
   - A. heart or inverted triangle
   - B. diamond
   - C. pear or triangle
   - D. hexagon

3. If a person's face has a lower zone that is rounded and wider than the upper and middle zones, they have which of the following face shapes?
   - A. heart or inverted triangle
   - B. diamond
   - C. pear or triangle
   - D. hexagon

4. Which two shapes are virtually the same except for the existence of a widow's peak at the hairline? (Circle two answers)
   - A. pear
   - B. inverted triangle
   - C. heart
   - D. triangle

5. Which shape indicates little or no cosmetic correction because of its structural similarity to the oval shape?
   - A. heart or inverted triangle
   - B. diamond
   - C. pear or triangle
   - D. hexagon

6. Refer to your drawing in Figure 2–17 in Chapter 2. Which of the following face shapes most resembles your face shape?
   - A. oval
   - B. long
   - C. square
   - D. round
   - E. heart or inverted triangle
   - F. diamond
   - G. pear or triangle
   - H. hexagon

(continues)

7. Identify the face shape of each face below. Each of the eight face shapes is represented.

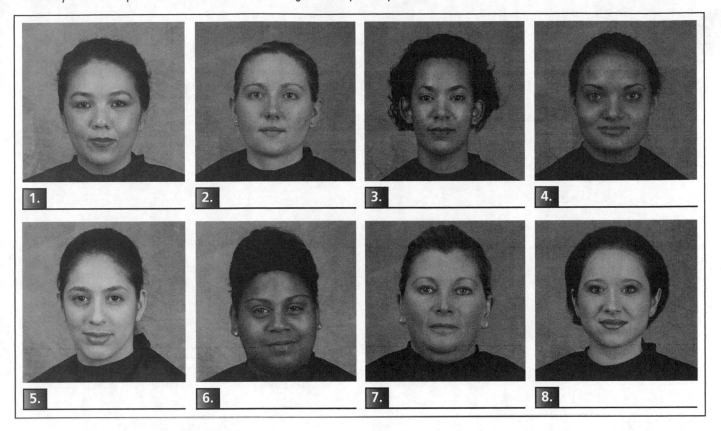

1.

2.

3.

4.

5.

6.

7.

8.

Summary—Face Shape Theory

You should now have a comfortable working knowledge of the different theories regarding face shapes and of the different face shapes themselves. You can choose to utilize face shape theory with any combination of different face shapes or decide to disregard it entirely. However, now your choice is an educated one and not one based on a lack of knowledge.

Possessing the ability to determine a client's face shape will assist you in performing corrective techniques more effectively. It will also assist you in choosing a client's optimal eyebrow shape as outlined in later chapters.

REFERENCES

D'Angelo, J., Lees, M., Dean, P. S., Miller, E., Dietz, S., Zani, A., & Hinds, C. 2003. *Milady's standard comprehensive training for estheticians.* Clifton Park, NY: Delmar Learning.

Gerson, J. (1999). *Milady's standard textbook for professional estheticians* (8th ed.). Clifton Park, NY: Delmar Learning.

Villa, L. P. (1987). *Cosmetology: The art of making up.* Toronto, Canada: Gage Educational Publishing Company.

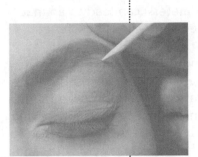

Chapter 4

THE STUDY OF EYE SET

Learning Objectives

After reading this chapter, you should be able to:

1. Name the three different eye sets.

2. Describe the one-eye rule.

3. Identify the primary measurement and the secondary consideration when determining the eye set of a client.

4. Discuss the two long-standing rules that prescribe ideal lip and base of the nose proportions.

5. Identify your eye set.

Tools you will need:

- a six-inch ruler
- pencil and paper

In this chapter, you will study the important task of determining a client's eye set. Eye set refers to how the eyes are situated in relation to the features of the face. The eye set is determined by understanding the width or narrowness of the eyes in relation to length and width of the nose and lips. Our discussion will incorporate many long-standing rules governing the ideal location of these three prominent facial features. Note that ideal facial proportions rarely exist on a person's face, but are used as a guideline to enhance the facial appearance. In later chapters, you will need to recall these guidelines when deciding which cosmetic corrections you wish to make to the client's eyebrows to visually balance other features of the face.

The One-Eye Rule

A long-standing principle that has guided the determination of eye set is that the distance between the eyes should be 3.5 centimeters or the width of one eye (Figure 4–1). The one-eye rule says that if the distance between a person's eyes is shorter than one eye width or less than 3.5 centimeters,

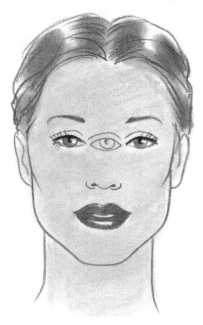

Figure 4–1.   The one-eye rule or the 3.5 cm rule

that person's eyes are close set. This rule is commonly used and can sometimes provide an accurate assessment of eye set. However, each person's facial measurements and eye size are quite different, so using a distance that measures the same amount for everyone (3.5 centimeters) can lead to an inaccurate assessment when contemplating eye set.

Instead, we recommend that the features of each person's face help determine the eye set. This method is more accurate as it takes into consideration relative focal points of the face—the nose and the lips—on which to base the assessment. It is also consistent with the other aspects of symmetry and facial balance, which are subscribed to in this book.

It should be mentioned that some beauty professionals merely "eyeball" whether a client has close-set, well-set, or wide-set eyes. Only in obvious cases can this be easily determined. However, a person's eye set is not always so obvious. In cases where the correct eye set is misconstrued, the necessary correction may be overlooked.

The Relational Measurement of Determining Eye Set

In order to correctly determine every client's eye set, it is necessary to make your assessment using the primary measurement along with the secondary consideration as described in detail below.

Primary Measurement

Use a straight-edged object such as a ruler. Place the ruler at the base of the nose, vertically upward.

- If the inner corner of the eye is inside the ruler, the person has close-set eyes with relation to the width of the base of the nose (Figure 4–2).

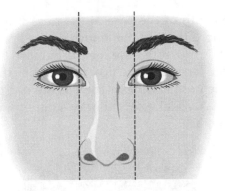

Figure 4–2.   Close-set eyes

- If the inner corner of the eye is directly in line with the ruler, the person has well-set eyes with relation to the width of the base of the nose (Figure 4–3).

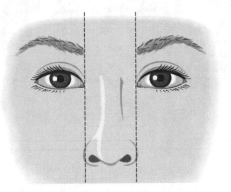

Figure 4–3.   Well-set eyes

- If the inner corner of the eye is outside the line of the ruler, the person has wide-set eyes with relation to the width of the base of the nose (Figure 4–4).

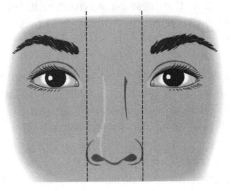

Figure 4–4.   Wide-set eyes

Secondary Consideration

The determination of eye set using the base of the nose as the primary indicator is always accurate. The secondary consideration, lip length, must be studied to ascertain whether or not to make the cosmetic correction as indicated by the initial eye set judgment.

For example, if a person's eyes are close set and their lips are narrow (see Figure 4–5), then one must consider whether or not to make a cosmetic correction to give the illusion of widening the eyes.

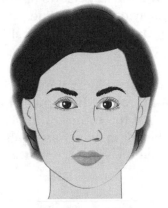

Figure 4–5.   Before—A woman with close-set eyes and narrow lips

Figure 4–6 shows the results of creating the illusion of widening the close-set eyes of a person who has narrow lips. Making the correction in this instance creates an imbalance in the facial appearance.

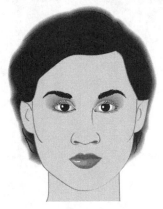

Figure 4–6.   After—An ineffective correction creates imbalance in this client's appearance

In considering whether or not to make cosmetic corrections in such cases, use the following rules regarding proportions of the lips and the nose to assist you in making these decisions.

The Rules Governing Ideal Proportions of the Nose and Lips

To determine whether a person's lips or base of the nose are unusually narrow or wide, consider the following long-standing rules of ideal facial proportions:

1. Hold a ruler vertically at the inside of the iris. It should pass through the corner of a relaxed lip (Figure 4–7). If the corner of the lip is inside the line, the lips may be narrow. If the lip corner is outside the vertical line, the lips may be wide.

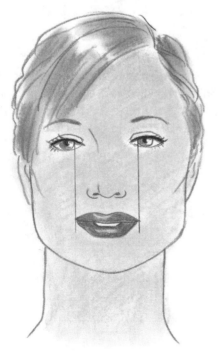

Figure 4–7.   Lip width test

2. The width of the base of the nose should be no more than $\frac{1}{2}$ the length of the lips (Figure 4–8). If the nose base measures more than $\frac{1}{2}$ of the length of the lips, then either the base of the nose is wide or the lips are narrow, or both. A visual assessment will determine which is the case.

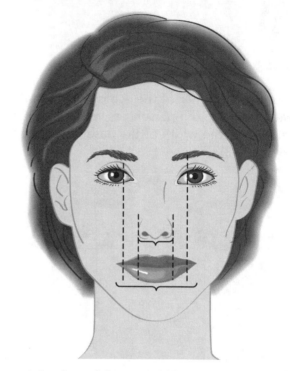

Figure 4–8.   Base of the nose width test

Again, the secondary consideration given to the lips does not change the eye set determination made using the base of the nose. Considering the lip length and the nose base width will help determine which cosmetic changes should or should not be made based on the eye set assessment.

The following practice sheet will teach you to study the relative positioning of the eyes, nose, and mouth so you can consistently evaluate the eye set of your clients. After you determine a client's eye set, you can apply corrective techniques to her eyebrows as outlined in Chapter 8. You will also be able to perform other cosmetic corrections to improve her overall appearance.

Practice Sheet for Determining Eye Set

Use the practice sheet to determine your own eye set.

STEP #1: Determination of Eye Set

Hold a ruler vertically at the base of the nose. If the inner corner of the eye falls: (check the appropriate line)

_____ inside the line of the ruler, then you have close-set eyes in relation to the width of the base of the nose.

_____ on the line of the ruler, then you have well-set eyes.

_____ outside the line of the ruler, then you have wide-set eyes.

STEP #2: Base of the Nose Width in Relation to Lip Length

Measure horizontally the width of the base of the nose: _____

Measure horizontally the length of a relaxed lip:

_____

Are the lips at least twice the width as the base of the nose? _____

_____

If not, then either the base of the nose is wide or the lips are narrow. Document your determination based on the measurements and a visual study of the face.

_____

_____

STEP #3: Lip Length with Respect to Eye Width

Hold a ruler vertically at the inner side of the iris. Does the corner of the lip fall inside, on, or outside the line of the ruler? _____

If inside, then the lips may be narrow or the eyes may be wide.

If "on," then the lips are well proportioned and the eyes and lips are balanced.

If outside, then the lips may be wide, the eyes may be narrow, or both.

Steps 2 and 3 will assist in deciding whether or not to make the cosmetic corrections as indicated by the eye set determination.

REFERENCES

D'Angelo, J., Lees, M., Dean, P. S., Miller, E., Dietz, S., Zani, A., & Hinds, C. 2003. *Milady's standard comprehensive training for estheticians.* Clifton Park, NY: Delmar Learning.

Villa, L. P. (1987). *Cosmetology: The art of making up.* Toronto, Canada: Gage Educational Publishing Company.

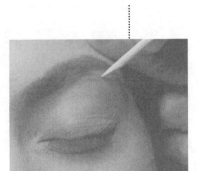

Chapter 5

ASSESSING THE FACIAL FEATURES

Learning Objectives

After reading this chapter, you should be able to:

1. List the 10 observable features of the face that determine cosmetic corrections and eyebrow placement.

2. Discuss how the ideal lip size and shape has evolved over the last few decades.

3. Describe how the overall style of the client may affect her preference in cosmetics and in eyebrow shape selection.

4. Specify the general rule of consistency regarding overall feature size in relation to eyebrow thickness.

5. Understand the concept of subjectivity with respect to cosmetic application and the selection of an optimal eyebrow shape and color.

6. Identify the main factor when deciding on the appropriate brow thickness for a client.

Tools you will need:

- fashion magazines
- ruler
- pen

In this chapter, you will focus on the analysis of the individual features of the face, which will strengthen your ability to perform successful "eyebrow design" work. As you learn to consider each feature, you will learn how to adapt the design to improve your clients' eyebrows and their overall appearance.

Once again, we must stress that a person's features will not always match the ideal standards in characteristic and proportion. Everyone's facial features are uniquely different with respect to size, shape, and location. These ideal standards are used to provide a benchmark for deciding which corrective techniques (cosmetic corrections) you may wish to perform.

After studying these foundational chapters, you will have a solid basis for making decisions in your capacity as a beauty professional. If you decide to adhere to or depart from a rule in certain instances, that decision will be based on a deliberate and educated opinion, not by accident or neglect.

Ten Facial Features to Assess

You will be able to provide your clients with the optimal hair, makeup, and eyebrow enhancement services when you make a complete assessment of their features. First, we will describe each of the 10 features. This will be followed by a section of practice worksheets requiring you to assess two models—yourself and someone of your choosing—and record your findings. Systematically assessing and recording this information will give you a clearer idea of what is and is not proportional. In your professional work, you will be able to accomplish this complete assessment without the use of the worksheets provided in this chapter. However, it is beneficial to use the worksheets as tools to train you to analyze specific parts of the face. The following 10 features will be analyzed.

1. Eye set
2. Eye size and orientation
3. Nose
4. Lips
5. Forehead
6. Chin
7. Hairstyle
8. Age
9. Overall style
10. Overall feature size

During this analysis of features, you will be consulting with clients to find out what they like and do not like about their facial characteristics. Gather information about how the clients usually wear their hair and makeup, and how they dress most days. This will help you understand their overall style.

Use soft, diplomatic words during the client consultation. Compliment positive characteristics. Be tactful when describing possibly less desirable ones. For example, instead of saying, "Your eyes are close set," you can describe how the eyes can be cosmetically enhanced to "make them look more dramatic."

Each feature resides in a specific facial zone or has an impact on one or more facial zones. Performing corrective techniques to the eyebrow to give the illusion of improving a feature will improve the appearance of its zone as well as the overall appearance.

We will revisit these 10 features again in Chapter 8 and learn how to perform the corrective techniques to enhance the clients' appearance.

Eye Set

As discussed at length in Chapter 4, it is imperative to distinguish the clients' eye set in order to choose the correct location for their eyebrows. Corrective changes to the beginning point of the eyebrow depend almost entirely on eye set.

To review the method for determining eye set, place a ruler vertically upward at the base of the nose. If the ruler is aligned with the inner corner of the eye, the eyes are well set. If the ruler goes through any part of the eye, the eyes are close set. If the eye is outside the ruler, the eyes are wide set.

Eye Size and Orientation

The determination of eye size can be accurately made based on a visual analysis. Look at the overall size of the client's head, the nose, and the lips to decide whether the client has small, medium, or large eyes. For example, Figure 5–1 shows a medium-sized face with a medium-sized nose, full lips, and small eyes. Figure 5–2 shows the same features, except for the eyes, which are large.

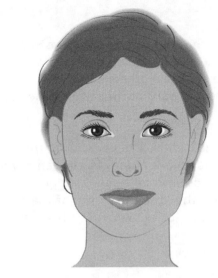

Figure 5–2.   Large eyes

Eye orientation can be distinguished as almond-shaped, even, or drooping. An almond-shaped eye ends slightly upward (Figure 5–3). An even eye has a beginning and ending that are on the same horizontal plane (Figure 5–4). A drooping eye has an ending point that is lower than its beginning point (Figure 5–5).

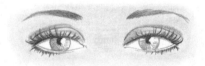

Figure 5–3.   Almond-shaped eyes

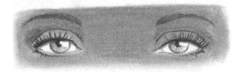

Figure 5–4.   Even eyes

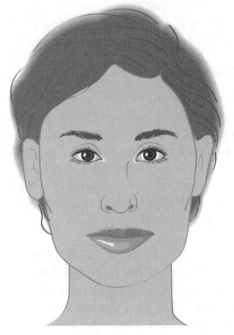

Figure 5–1.   Small eyes

Figure 5–5.   Drooping eyes

The Nose

Each nose is uniquely different (Figure 5–6). Some are thin while others are wide. Some have a small point at the tip while others have a ball-shaped tip. Some have downward nostrils while other gently turn upward.

Be careful and gentle when discussing the characteristics of your client's nose. More than any other feature, the nose can be a source of good and bad emotions. It is the absolute center of the face and one of the most noticeable and visible features.

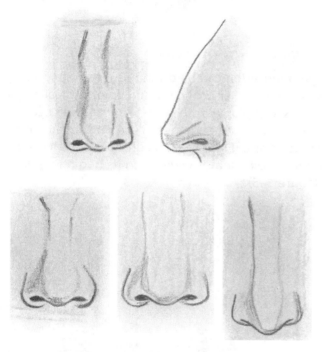

Figure 5–6. The many different characteristics of the nose make each unique

When analyzing the nose, make a visual assessment of the following qualities:

- overall size: small, medium, or large
- bridge width: wide, medium, or narrow
- bridge length: long, medium, or short
- bridge traits: hook, bump, gentle slope, or up-ward turn

- base of the nose: wide, medium, or narrow
- tip of the nose: pointy, ball-shaped, or other
- nostrils: visible or not visible (frontal, nonsmiling glance)

The Lips

The ideal size and proportion of the lips has changed over the past few decades. Previously, women's lips were thought to be ideal if the top lip was smaller than the bottom lip, and the lip was small to medium in size. The more recent standard, which can be seen by glancing through fashion magazines, is a large, full lip. This new lip size has become the standard of beauty and sexuality in our culture, so much so that some women are having collagen injected into their lips to achieve a fuller lip appearance.

Analyze the following qualities of the lips:

- overall lip size: thin, medium, full
- is the upper lip smaller than the lower lip? Yes/No
- are the lips in proportion with the width of the base of the nose (is the base of the nose 1/2 the length of the lips)? Yes/No
- are the lips in proportion with the width of the eyes (this is a visual assessment)? Yes/No

The Forehead and the Chin

The forehead has many different characteristics that can have a major impact on a person's appearance. The forehead characteristics often dictate the type of hairstyle worn by a client. For example, if a person has an attractive forehead, she will often wear her hair pulled back off the face and her hair is likely to be all one layer; if it is layered, it is usually worn without bangs.

When a woman has a wide, deep, or otherwise prominent forehead, her hairstyle will usually include bangs, layers, and some type of cover for the top and sides of her forehead. You will assess a client's hairstyle, along with her other features because of the impact each feature has on the other.

With respect to the forehead, take note of the following characteristics. Remember to pull the hair back completely from the face when studying these characteristics.

- forehead breadth: narrow, medium, or prominent
- hairline shape: horizontal from ear to ear, rounded, pointed, or oval
- is there a widow's peak? Yes/No

The chin can have many different characteristics as well. Yet having a memorable and prominent chin occurs less often than with other features of the face. Still, it is necessary to take note of the characteristics of the chin and define its impact on the lower zone and the overall facial appearance.

Study the following characteristics of the chin:

- the depth of the chin: receding, protruding, or in line with the jaw
- shape of the chin: pointed, rounded, flat, or other

Hairstyle

A person's hairstyle choices with regard to color, style, and length greatly impact her overall appearance. Because of this, remember to consider these three questions when studying the hairstyle selections of your clients.

1. How does the hairstyle complement the overall style? Overall style helps dictate the selection of a pleasing eyebrow shape during the "eyebrow design" process, as well as other cosmetic choices made by and on behalf of the client.
2. Does the current hairstyle complement the client's face shape and dimensions? For example, a client with an inverted triangle-shaped face may be wearing a hairstyle that parts in the middle and exposes the wide upper zone. A more appealing style might include cutting the hair to create bangs to soften the edges of the hairline, making the upper zone appear smaller. Just because a client has "always worn

it that way" doesn't mean that it is the best style for her features.
3. Is the brow shape and thickness consistent with the client's haircolor and style? If a client has light blond hair and wears it in a soft, curly style, it would be inconsistent to have very dark, thick, severely arched eyebrows.

Consider the following elements regarding your client's hair:

- is the hair always worn pulled back completely from the face? Yes/No
- hair length: short, medium, or long
- hair consistency: straight, wavy, or curly
- bangs? Yes/No
- haircolor(s)

The Effects of Age

One must consider the age of the client when contemplating any new beauty enhancement in hairstyle, haircolor, skin care, and makeup. The eyebrow shape, thickness, and color chosen for an older client will be much different from that chosen for a younger client. Generally, a younger client can wear the latest "fad" in clothing and makeup and look wonderful. Older clients will likely have better results if they allow their features, age, and style to dictate what choices they make.

Also with aging comes a gradual downward movement of the features. As a beauty professional, you can assist clients by cosmetically enhancing their features to provide a nonsurgical lift to their appearance. For example, choosing an eyebrow shape with an ending point that is higher than the beginning point will give the appearance of lifting the client's eyes.

Finally, aging affects the color and texture of the eyebrows, the skin, and the hair. All of this should be considered during the consultation process.

Consider the following questions with regard to the age of the client:

- chronological or approximate age
- signs of aging around the eyes: minimal or wrinkling
- are there gray hairs in the eyebrow? Yes/No
- have the eyebrows been colored? Yes/No
- can the client grow brow hairs in the sparse areas? Yes/No

Overall Style or Personality Type

A person's overall style affects cosmetic selections just as a person's cosmetic selections affect overall style. As people make hair and makeup choices, they often do so within the boundaries of their overall style, which can be categorized as their "personality type."

Consider the following personality types:

- conservative
- artistic
- flamboyant and extravagant
- relaxed and carefree
- intense or type A
- demure
- natural

This list is by no means exhaustive and can be written using any number of personality types. The point is that you will want to be consistent with people's overall image when choosing their eyebrow shape. Determining the client's personality type will help you do so.

As you begin the practice of defining your client's personality type, you will notice common grooming habits for the women in each category. Beauty professionals often do this instinctively. For example, conservative women will maintain certain hairstyles that will look remarkably different from those worn by relaxed, carefree women. A person's makeup routine is also consistent with personality type. An artistic person is likely to wear more dramatic colors, with a heavier application of makeup, whereas a natural personality type is likely to wear little or no makeup.

A classic eyebrow shape that is medium to thick and that requires minimal hair removal will look best on a natural personality type. This person would look inconsistent with a high fashion, heavily filled in eyebrow. On the other hand, if a person is extravagant, they may look best in a highly arched, made-up eyebrow. Understanding your client's overall style or personality type will guide you in helping your clients make optimal hair, makeup, and "eyebrow design" choices.

Overall Feature Size

Overall feature size is the main factor when considering the best eyebrow thickness for your client. The rule of consistency suggests that a person's features should be of the same relative size to achieve a balanced appearance. If they are not, you can apply cosmetics to create the illusion of consistency among the features.

The rule of consistency as applied to eyebrow shape selection suggests that a person with delicate features should maintain a brow that is thin or barely medium in thickness (Figure 5–7). A per-

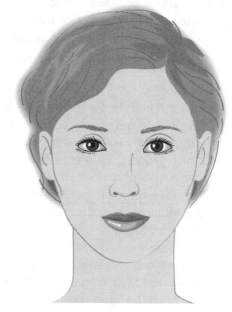

Figure 5–7. Small, delicate features look more consistent with a thinner eyebrow

son who has larger overall features should maintain a brow that is medium or thick (Figure 5–8).

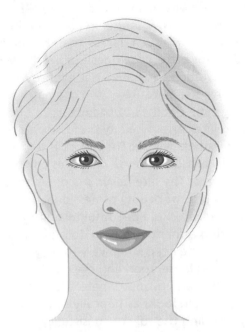

Figure 5–8.   Large, strong features are more balanced with a medium or thick eyebrow

Reggie Wells, longtime makeup artist for Oprah Winfrey and many other famous Hollywood faces, agrees. In his book entitled *Face Painting*, Mr. Wells writes, "If you have a very full or wide eye, for example, your brow should be full, not thin. If you have small eyes, you should thin your brows so they don't overwhelm the eye area and detract from the beauty of the eye itself."

While analyzing a client's overall feature size, focus on the following elements:

- size of the eyes: small, medium, or large
- size of the nose: small, medium, or large
- size of the lips: small, medium, or large
- length of face: _____ inches
- width of face: _____ inches
- shape (or shapes) of face: _____ _____ _____
- head size: small, medium, or large

Breaking the Rules

Once you understand and utilize this rule of consistency, you will learn when it is appropriate to bend or break it. The following are examples of breaking this rule and still providing the client with outstanding results.

1. When clients are young, they can wear the latest eyebrow fashion trends regardless of their feature size. Youthfulness can hide many beauty and fashion mistakes, including hairstyle, clothing, and makeup choices. An example of how youthfulness can hide a less than desirable choice is shown in the following photographs. The photograph in Figure 5–9 shows

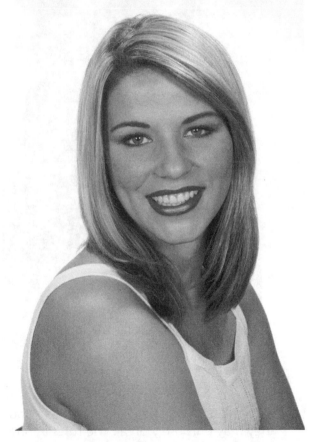

Figure 5–9.   Medium/large features with a thin eyebrow

a young woman wearing a thin eyebrow shape. The photograph in Figure 5–10 shows the same woman wearing an eyebrow that is medium in thickness. The medium eyebrow shape follows the rule of consistency. Her features include large, beautiful eyes, a medium-sized nose, and large, full lips. The medium-sized eyebrow is more consistent with her overall appearance. Most professionals would agree that the medium eyebrow looks better on her. Yet because of current trends, her age, and her beauty, she can wear the thin shape and still look wonderful.

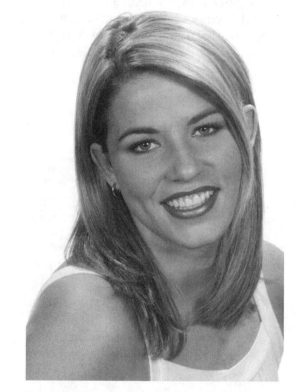

Figure 5–10.   Following the rule of consistency, medium/large-sized features with an eyebrow of medium thickness

2. If clients have a certain reputation or "look," they may purposely break the rules in order to achieve that look. Pamela Anderson provides a good example. She has large eyes and large, full lips. Following the rule of consistency, she should choose a medium to thick eyebrow shape. However, she wears a very thin, high-fashion eyebrow shape. In addition, her eyebrow color is much darker than her hair color. This color difference does not work well on most women. However, her eyebrows work well for her because of the dramatic and edgy image she chooses to project.

3. There are certain beauty professionals who have pure esthetic vision. Their work is derived from a wholly artistic point of view. This type of individual is rare. The late Kevyn Aucoin is an example of this type of beauty professional. His book, *Making Faces*, is a beautiful testimony to his amazing esthetic talent. In doing his mother's makeup, Kevyn chose a very thin eyebrow. His mom has large, sparkling eyes, a strong nose and chin, and proportionately full lips. However, Mrs. Aucoin looks esthetically attractive despite his bending the rule of consistency.

4. While many clients give the beauty professional creative license to enhance their appearance, some clients come to the salon with absolute and definitive opinions regarding what results they desire. It is likely that you have encountered this type of client who wants a high arch when a flatter brow shape would better suit her features or who demands blond hair when her natural color is the darkest brown. This client may be best served by giving her the look that she wants. Note that your client may not have "outstanding results" according to your standards, but if she does according to her standards, then you will have made your client very happy and pleased with her appearance.

The following practice sheet provides you with guidelines for studying the specific features of the face. After completing this exercise, you will be confident in your appraisal of your client's facial features, and, in turn, you will be confident in your decisions to make or not make various cosmetic corrections to those features.

Facial Feature Analysis Worksheets

Suggested Use: Complete the feature analysis on yourself. Photocopy this blank form and perform a second feature analysis on another person or student. Compare the results. This activity provides important practice in analyzing facial features.

Facial Feature Analysis of: _____

Performed by: _____

Date: _____

1. Eye set is _____ close, well, wide

2. Eye size is _____ small, medium, large

3. Eye orientation is _____ almond, even, drooping

4. Nose size is _____ small, medium, large

5. Bridge width is _____ wide, medium, narrow

6. Bridge length is _____ long, medium, short

7. Bridge traits _____ hook, bump, upward turn, other

8. Base of nose _____ wide, medium, narrow

9. Tip of nose _____ pointy, ball-shaped, other

10. Nostrils _____ visible or not visible (front glance, nonsmiling)

11. Lip size _____ thin, medium, full

12. Upper lip smaller than lower lip? _____ Yes/No

13. Lips in proportion with base of nose? _____ Yes/No

14. Lips in width-wise proportion to eyes? _____ Yes/No

15. Forehead breadth _____ narrow, medium, prominent

16. Hairline shape _____ rounded, pointed, oval, flat (ear-to-ear)

17. Widow's peak? _____ Yes/No

18. Hairstyle _____down, pulled back

19. Hair length_____short, medium, long

20. Hair consistency _____straight, wavy, curly

21. Bangs? _____ Yes/No

22. Haircolor (s) _____

23. Age _____

24. Personality type _____ conservative, natural, artistic, other

REFERENCES

Aucoin, K. (1997). *Making faces.* New York: Little, Brown and Company.

D'Angelo, J., Lees, M., Dean, P. S., Miller, E., Dietz, S., Zani, A., & Hinds, C. 2003. *Milady's standard comprehensive training for estheticians.* Clifton Park, NY: Delmar Learning.

Villa, L. P. (1987). Cosmetology: *The art of making up.* Toronto, Canada: Gage Educational Publishing Company.

Wells, R. (1998). *Face painting.* New York: Henry Holt and Company.

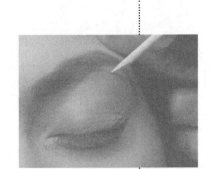

Chapter 6

ASSESSING THE EYEBROW

Learning Objectives

After reading this chapter, you should be able to:

1. List the four features of the eyebrow that should be analyzed.

2. Describe what you will determine about the eyebrow for each of the four characteristics.

3. Describe how to trim the eyebrow hairs.

4. Name three things you will learn when you assess the texture of eyebrow hair.

5. List possible color choices for an eyebrow fill-in based on hair and brow color.

6. Define two types of excess eyebrow hair.

7. Describe how you would help a client decide if tuft hairs should be removed.

Tools you will need:

- eyebrow brush/comb
- small scissors or cuticle nippers
- brow setting gel
- eyebrow pencils or powders in a wide array of colors including dark brown, medium brown, light brown, taupe, light auburn, dark auburn, yellow, and gray
- ruler
- fashion or beauty magazines

The assessment of the eyebrow follows the assessment of the facial features. As you gain experience, you can perform the two assessments simultaneously. Eventually, you will be able to make both assessments in approximately five to ten minutes.

During your analysis of the eyebrows, ask clients what they like and do not like about their eyebrows. Your primary goal is to learn what the client wants, so gather as much information as possible to achieve both the result desired by the client and a result that is esthetically correct.

Table 6–1 lists the four characteristics of the brow you will analyze and what you will determine for each.

The purpose, tools, and procedures for each feature are discussed below. This step of analyzing the characteristics of the eyebrow will prepare you and your client for the "eyebrow design" and hair removal processes.

Assess the Length

Long, unruly, or curly eyebrows that extend beyond the lines of the eyebrow shape look unkempt and detract from a person's appearance. Look through any fashion or trade magazine and you will notice that the eyebrows of models are clean, without long or straggly hairs. Just the small step of trimming the brows makes a remarkable difference in appearance.

Purpose

To decide if trimming is necessary in order to clean up the eyebrow area and prepare the eyebrow for shaping.

Tools

- brow brush/comb
- small scissors or cuticle nippers

Procedure

Using the comb side of the eyebrow brush, comb the brows upward and outward. Starting at the beginning point of the eyebrow, comb the brow upward and stop the motion as the comb reaches the uppermost part of the brow. Hold the comb in place. Note any hairs that appear excessively long. If none of the hairs appear excessively long or if all brow hairs are within the eyebrow shape after the comb is released and the brows hairs are settled, then they are the proper length and do not need to be trimmed. If that is the case, then you will move to the next assessment. If you determine that

TABLE 6–1.   ANALYSIS OF EYEBROW FEATURES

Assess the:	To determine:
Length of individual brow hairs	If trimming is necessary
Texture of the eyebrow hairs	If a brow setting product should be used
Color and tone of the brow hairs	What color(s) and tone(s) of powder or pencil can be used for fill-in
Excess eyebrow hair	Whether tuft hairs should or should not be removed, and to decide which type of hair removal will be performed

the hairs require trimming, proceed to trim them as described below.

Divide the length of the brow into thirds with imaginary lines. Begin with the first third that is closest to the inner corner. Comb the brow and hold the comb in place just above the brow line (Figure 6–1). Trim the brow hairs using small scissors or nippers so they are approximately three millimeters longer than the top of the brow line. Perform the trimming while holding the brows upward in the comb. Move to the next section of the brow and repeat the procedure until the entire eyebrow has been trimmed. Go back to the beginning point, and using the brush side, brush the eyebrow to see how the hairs lie. If the brow is clean and the hairs are in place, then the length is appropriate. If specific hairs appear too long, trim them again, only one millimeter at a time.

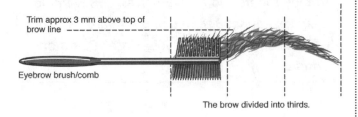
Trim approx 3 mm above top of brow line
Eyebrow brush/comb
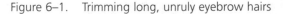
The brow divided into thirds.

Figure 6–1.   Trimming long, unruly eyebrow hairs

Be very careful during the trimming of the brow hairs. If they are cut too short, they will no longer lay flat but stick straight out from the face. It is better to cut only a little bit at a time, even if the process takes longer.

Assess the Texture

Purpose

To discern brow hair texture and hair growth pattern to decide if a setting gel is necessary, and to assist in determining the optimal eyebrow shape by studying the existing arch and shape of the brow.

Tools

- eyebrow brush/comb
- clean fingertips
- brow setting product for use later in the process

Procedure

Brush Test: Use the brush side of the brush/comb and brush the eyebrows in place. Pause. While you are consulting with the client, notice if the brow hairs move or if they stay in place. If the client's brows do not stay in place, then a brow setting product should be used.

Fingertip Test: Touch one of the brows with clean fingertips to discern the texture. The texture can range from fine and soft to thick and wiry or bristle-like. The more wiry the brow, the more likely they are to stay in place. However, if a wiry brow grows in an erratic, undesirable direction, then a brow setting product can be used to align hairs, giving a well-groomed look.

Decide whether the client should use a brow-setting product based on the brush test and the fingertip test. Hair spray is not recommended for use in setting the brow hairs because it almost always contains alcohol that can irritate the skin.

Take notice of the direction of the growth of the hairs. Ideally, the brow hairs will grow upward and outward (Figure 6–2).

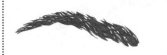 

Figure 6–2.   Eyebrow hairs growing upward and outward

Some of the more difficult cases occur when all or most of the hairs grow downward (Figure 6–3). A good brow setting product can help remedy this problem.

Figure 6–3.   Downward growth of eyebrow hairs

Finally, examine the eyebrow closely to see where the existing high point or arch is. Oftentimes, the client's eyebrow will appear flatter than it really is. This occurs when brow hair at the arch is sparse (Figure 6–4). Eyebrow hairs at the highest part of the brow are often sparse and grow downward. With only light fill-in in that area, you can make a remarkable difference by highlighting the existing arch and giving clients the lift they desire. Figures 6–4 and 6–5 show the exact same eyebrow except that the eyebrow in Figure 6–5 has had the arch area filled in where it was previously sparse.

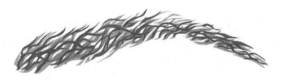

Figure 6–4.   Before—This eyebrow appears flat because existing brow hairs at the arch are sparse.

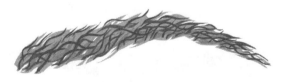

Figure 6–5. After—Same exact brow shape as in Figure 6–4 except the existing arch hairs are filled in and the arch is defined.

In addition to using fill-in to alter and/or enhance the color of the eyebrows, you may choose to talk to your client about tinting. Tinting is a method of darkening the color of the brows using chemicals that are safe around the eyes. Tinting is discussed in detail in Chapter 12. Each state's Cosmetology Board provides regulations regarding safe tinting ingredients and procedures. It is essential to check those regulations before providing the tinting service.

The individual state Boards of Cosmetology in all of the fifty states do not allow professionals in the salon to use haircolor or bleach to change the color of the brows. Unfortunately, some professionals provide this service at a great risk to their clients and to themselves. This warning bears repeating: Before going forward with any of these options, consult your state's Board of Cosmetology.

Assess the Eyebrow Hair Color

The choice of fill-in color is based on the color and tone of the client's hair, skin, and brows. Choosing fill-in color is both an objective and a subjective decision. It is based on the esthetic point of view of the professional and the client, coupled with some sensible color guidelines. Choosing an attractive fill-in color is as important as choosing the correct brow shape. If the color is not appealing to the client, she will not be happy with the end result.

Purpose

The purpose of the color assessment is to make sure that the hair and brow colors are complementary, and to choose fill-in colors that look attractive on the client. One of the main benefits of filling in the brow with powder or pencil is that the brows can be made symmetrical. Fill-in can also change the shape of the brow, as well as ensure that it is the proper and most flattering length.

Tools

- the following charts and tips
- eyebrow powders and/or pencils in a wide array of colors including dark brown, medium brown, light brown, taupe, gray, yellow, dark auburn, and light auburn

Procedure

First, decide whether the existing brow color works well with the client's hair color, skin color, and skin tone. If the existing brow color is agreeable, then match the pencil or powder color to the existing brow color. If a color change is desired, decide whether to subtly change the color with powder or pencil, or to tint the client's eyebrows. If the client decides to have her brows tinted, that service should be done 24 hours after the hair removal service is performed. If the client insists on using haircolor or bleach to change the brow color, explain that she must perform that procedure at home because you are not allowed to perform bleaching or haircoloring to the brows in the salon.

Second, make sure that the color tone (temperature) of the powder or pencil is consistent with the client's hair and skin tones. Eyebrow makeup, like all other makeup, has warm, cool, or neutral tones. Warm colors have an orange or yellow undertone, while cool colors have a gray or blue undertone. (For a thorough explanation of color theory, refer to *Milady's Standard Comprehensive Training for Estheticians* textbook.) Colors that have a neutral tone can be used on both warm- and cool-toned skin and hair. For example, there are some neutral taupe shades that can be used for all women and appear to blend in, regardless of whether they have warm or cool undertones. Certain auburn powders

can exhibit this neutral tendency, appearing more orange when worn on a warm-toned person and more burgundy when worn on a cool-toned person. Other colors are not neutral and take on and create a definite warmth or coolness. Applying the incorrect color tone to the brow can create poor results whereas choosing shades with complementary color tones can create outstanding results.

To review, the process of fill-in color selection requires the following steps:

1. Decide whether the existing brow color should be chemically changed.
2. Match the existing or newly tinted brow color with fill-in colors that have a similar or slightly lighter color and tone.

To assist you in deciding which colors to experiment with and use on a client, refer to Table 6–2, which lists brow color options based on the client's hair and eyebrow color.

The following is a list of tips for choosing an appropriate fill-in color.

1. "Matching" the eyebrow color can be done in different ways. Some experts believe that brow fill-in color(s) should be a shade lighter than the existing brow color. Others say to match the color as closely as possible. Either way is acceptable as long as the client is pleased with the results. The challenge with matching the fill-in color to the brow color is that the result can sometimes be too dark or severe. To avoid this, we recommend blending colors together and/or using other methods to lighten the appearance after the fill-in has been done. Both of these options are discussed below.

    Blending two or more colors together will help you achieve a better match, and hence a more natural looking eyebrow. Too often, beauty professionals rely on cosmetic manufacturers to provide the exact shade of powder that is needed. Mixing colors together puts the

Table 6–2. Brow Color Fill-in Suggestions

Hair Color	Brow Color	Brow Powder or Pencil Colors Mix and Blend for the Closest Match
Blonde	Blonde	Taupe, yellow
Blonde	Light brown	Light brown, taupe, yellow
Blonde	Dark brown	Medium brown, light brown, taupe, yellow
Blonde	Light auburn	Light brown, taupe, light auburn
Strawberry blonde	Strawberry blonde	Light auburn, taupe
Light brown/light auburn	Light brown	Light brown, light auburn, taupe, yellow
Medium ash brown/ Medium golden brown	Medium brown	Medium brown, light brown, taupe, gray
Medium auburn/ dark auburn	Medium auburn/ dark auburn	Dark, medium, and light brown, dark auburn, light auburn
Dark ash brown	Dark brown	Dark, medium, and light brown, taupe, gray, yellow
Black	Dark brown	Dark, medium, and light brown, taupe, gray
Black	Black	Dark brown, taupe, gray. Use black in rare cases
Gray	Gray, light brown	Light brown, taupe, gray

artistry in the hands of the professional and helps achieve a more dimensional look, much the way blending colors does for haircoloring.

There are two ways to make the fill-in look lighter. The first is to use either a pencil or an artist's brush with wet powder to draw in hair-like strokes. This way is preferred if the client wears little or no makeup. The second is to fill in the eyebrows using dry powder and an eyebrow powder applicator. After applying the brow setting gel, you can lightly powder the entire eyebrow using a light shade of pressed powder or eyebrow powder.

2. Taupe is considered a universal fill-in color because many taupe shades are neutral. It can be used on different brow colors, either alone or mixed with other fill-in colors.

3. Black eyebrow powder or pencil should rarely be used because it can appear too harsh and severe. Try a blend of the browns and taupe or gray first.

4. Some women's skin turns their makeup orange. If a pink blush is applied to this type of skin, it will turn to a coral (orangey) pink. If this happens, warm colors or neutral colors that have an orange undertone should not be applied. Instead, use a light or medium gray color by itself.

5. When you fill in the bare spots of an eyebrow to create symmetry, it is important to realize

that the overall look will be darker. That is because you are used to seeing skin color that you will be replacing with brow powder or pencil. Discuss this with the client during the consultation so she is prepared for the change. Lighten the fill-in colors as needed.

6. Eyebrow pencils contain wax. Therefore, pencil does not ordinarily stay on as long as a good powder. Try using powder to help your clients fill in their eyebrows, even if you and they are unaccustomed to doing so. The look you can achieve and the staying power of the powder will please both you and your client. Again, refer to a fashion magazine to see examples of fill-in to help you decide which result you prefer.

Assess Excess Eyebrow Hair

Two types of excess eyebrow hair are stubble hair and tuft hair (Figure 6-6). Stubble hair is excess eyebrow hair that is short and coarse, and is the regrowth from previously removed hairs. Tuft hair is excess eyebrow hair that grows straight upward. It exists at the inner corner of the eyebrow and is most often inside the optimal beginning point.

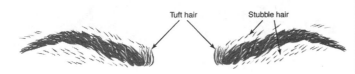

Figure 6–6.   Tuft hair and stubble hair

Purpose

There are two purposes in examining excess eyebrow hair. The first is to study the tuft and stubble hairs to decide if they should be removed during the hair removal process. The second is to help the client decide which type or types of hair removal she will choose after the "eyebrow design" process is complete.

Tools

- ruler
- eyebrow brush/comb
- skin-colored concealer

Procedure

First, locate any tuft hair that may exist. If you find eyebrow hairs that are growing straight up, then hold a ruler to the inner corner of the client's eye. Notice if the tuft hair is inside the ruler (Figure 6–7). This tuft hair is not part of the body of the eyebrow, and whether or not it is removed is subject to the client consultation. If the tuft hair is at the point of or to the outside of the ruler, it is part of the body of the eyebrow (Figure 6–8) and it must not be removed.

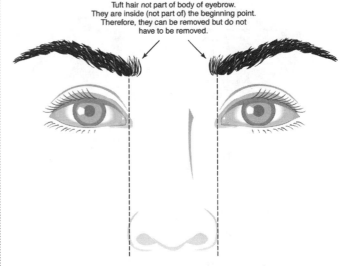

Tuft hair *not part of body of eyebrow.*
They are inside (not part of) the beginning point.
Therefore, they can be removed but do not have to be removed.

Figure 6–7.   Tuft hairs that are not part of the body of the brow can be removed

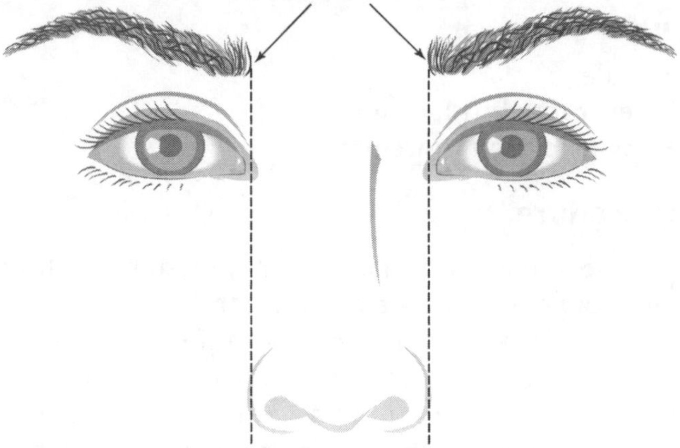

Tuft hairs that are part of the body of the eyebrow. They are outside the beginning point measurement line, and are, therefore, the beginning point of the eyebrow. Do not remove these tuft hairs.

Figure 6–8.   Tuft hairs that are part of the body of the brow should not be removed

To assist in deciding if the tuft hair that is not part of the body of the brow should be removed, you can use concealing makeup to temporarily cover those excess hairs. Have the client look in the mirror after the concealing makeup is applied. If she prefers the look of the brow without the tuft hair, she may choose to have it removed. Counsel your client and explain that many women have tuft hair; some decide to leave it while others decide to have it removed. Explain that removing it carries the obligation to continue to have it removed.

Next, examine the stubble hair that is outside the body of the eyebrow—both above and below the eyebrow—taking notice of the length and amount. Based on the characteristics of the stubble and tuft hair, you can help the client determine the best option for eyebrow hair removal. Chapter 11 provides an in-depth study of hair removal options. As you will learn in this later chapter, the client's decision regarding the choice of a preferred hair removal method is based on hair length and amount, cost, permanence, and other factors. Table 11–2 in Chapter 11 provides a comparative list of elements to consider when choosing a method of eyebrow hair removal. Use this table to assist you and your client in making the hair removal decision.

Practice Sheet for Assessing the Eyebrow—Length, Texture, Color, and Excess Eyebrow Hair

Practice the following steps on a classmate or a volunteer client.

Step #1: Assess the length of the brow hairs. Is trimming necessary? _____

Step #2: Assess the texture.

Describe the texture of the eyebrow. _____

Do the hairs appear to shift or stay in place? _____

Does the hair grow upward and outward or downward? _____

Will the client need a brow setting product? _____

Examine the eyebrow to locate its highest point.

Is the hair sparse at the location of the arch? _____

Does the hair at the arch grow upward or downward? _____

Step #3: Assess the Color

What is the client's eyebrow color? _____

What is the client's hair color? _____

What is the client's color tone (warm/cool)? _____

What colors will you blend together for this client's fill-in? _____

Experiment with powders and pencils to find a close match for fill-in.

Step #4: Assess the Excess Hair

Does the client have stubble hair? _____

What is the approximate length of the stubble hair? _____

Does the client have tuft hair? _____

If yes, is the tuft hair in between the brows or is it part of the eyebrow? _____

Will you remove the tuft hair? If so, how did you arrive at that decision? _____

Step #5: What type of hair removal of the eyebrows will you recommend for this client and why?

(Consider length of hair and amount of hair to be removed, among other factors.) _____

_____

_____

REFERENCES

D'Angelo, J., Lees, M., Dean, P. S., Miller, E., Dietz, S., Zani, A., & Hinds, C. 2003. *Milady's standard comprehensive training for estheticians.* Clifton Park, NY: Delmar Learning.

RULES OF PROPER EYEBROW MANAGEMENT

Learning Objectives

After reading this chapter, you should be able to:

1. Name six characteristics of the eyebrow that determine its shape.

2. Describe how to locate the ideal beginning point and ending point for the eyebrow.

3. Discuss the choice between an angled brow and a rounded brow.

4. Specify how to measure for the optimal eyebrow length.

5. Discuss why there is no standard for arch placement.

6. Give the term synonymous for "arch."

7. Describe the three alternatives for an eyebrow's ending point.

Tools you will need:

- ruler
- pen
- fashion or beauty magazines
- soft tape measure

Thus far, we have thoroughly studied the facial zones, face shapes, and eye set. We have also looked at the steps involved in assessing the facial features and have learned to perform an initial analysis of the eyebrows. The two bodies of knowledge you will learn in this chapter and the next are:

- the rules of proper eyebrow placement, guidelines specifically related to six elements that dictate shape selection and optimal eyebrow location
- corrective techniques to the eyebrows, a process of making cosmetic changes to the eyebrows to create the illusion of correcting undesired characteristics of the face, which relate to the 10 facial features studied in Chapter 5.

While Chapters 7 and 8 are interrelated, it is helpful to initially study them as a two-step process. You will often choose an initial eyebrow shape based on the guidelines, and then, while applying corrective techniques, alter the initial shape. As you gain experience, you will find that you will be applying the rules and the corrective techniques simultaneously.

The Rules of Proper Eyebrow Placement

An eyebrow shape can be broken down into six elements. Each element was developed based on guidelines that have evolved over time as professionals studied the best methods to bring balance and symmetry to the face. We will refer to these guidelines for selecting the initial brow shape and location as the rules of proper eyebrow placement. The following are the six elements of an eyebrow shape.

1. Beginning point
2. Arch
3. Ending point
4. Arched or rounded eyebrow shape

5. Eyebrow length
6. Open or closed ending point

The Beginning Point

The beginning point for the eyebrow is based on the location of the inner corner of the eye (Figure 7–1). Hold a ruler vertically at the inner corner of the eye. Where it intersects the line of the eyebrow is where the beginning point of the eyebrow should be. This beginning point may be moved slightly inward or outward during the corrective techniques assessment. You will learn about this and other corrections in the next chapter.

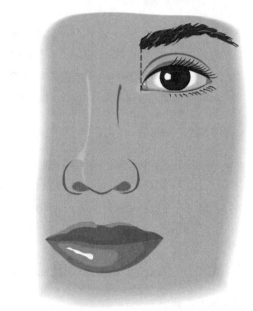

Figure 7–1.   The beginning point of the eyebrow

Recall from Chapter 6 that tuft hairs may be inside the vertical line or they may be part of the body of the eyebrow, and that removal of tuft hairs is partially dependent on where they are located. Also, you will find that some clients have removed eyebrow hair so there is no longer any hair at the beginning point where there should be. If that has occurred, it will be necessary to fill in that area with powder or pencil. Hopefully, the brow hair that is missing will grow back. If not, daily fill-in or permanent makeup may be necessary.

The Arch

The arch of the eyebrow is also known as the high point. In Chapter 6, you learned to locate and analyze the existing high point of the eyebrow during the examination of eyebrow texture. You learned to focus on that area to find the very highest part of the brow, regardless of whether brow hairs are sparse or full there. It is each client's existing arch that will provide you with the best guideline for enhancing or minimizing that facet. This is true because there is no accurate, definitive rule regarding the optimal location for the arch.

Some professionals support the notion that the arch should be directly above the outer rim of the iris. While this guideline is often used, it is not always accurate.

To verify this, take a moment and look at a women's magazine to visually confirm that optimal arch placement varies from person to person and is not consistently found in one place. For this purpose, study the photographs only of models that are looking straight on or at the camera. Place a ruler at the outer rim of the iris and notice where the high point is in relation to the iris. Test this on several models. You will see that the arch on models with well-designed eyebrows is located in many different places relative to the iris of the eye.

If you have a client who has only a few or no eyebrow hairs, you will need to rely on your esthetic ability and your technical knowledge to place the client's arch. You can also utilize information presented in Chapter 9 that provides suggested brow shapes for each face shape.

The Ending Point

The ending point of the eyebrow is easy to determine and its position should rarely be changed. Place a ruler at the base of the nose and hold the ruler diagonally so it intersects the outer corner of the eye and extends beyond it to the eyebrow. The ending point should be where the ruler intersects the eyebrow (Figure 7–2). Adhering to this rule gives the face the balance it needs, and prevents the eyebrow from being too long or too short for the other features of the face.

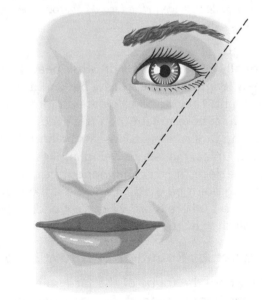

Figure 7–2.   The ending point of the eyebrow

As women grow older, the hairs on the outer half of their brow tend to become sparse or nonexistent because their hair regrowth slows. Overtweezing in the wrong location can also cause the brow hairs to become sparse. Regardless of whether hair exists in that area, the ending point should extend to where the ruler intersects the brow line (Figure 7–3).

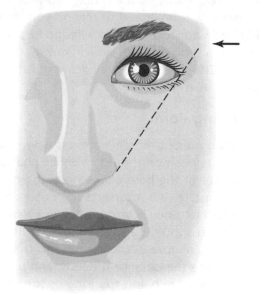

Figure 7–3.   Extending the eyebrow to the correct ending point will provide balance to the face. The arrow indicates where the ending point should be.

Occasionally, makeup artists or other beauty professionals lengthen the eyebrow beyond its correct ending point. They do so to create a more dramatic look. If you choose to lengthen the eyebrow, realize that the face is likely to lose its balanced appearance. Unless makeup is being applied for stage or special effects, it is recommended that the correct ending point be used. In addition, there are no circumstances where a brow's correct ending point should be shortened.

Arched versus Rounded Eyebrow Shape

In cases where the frame of the face is either overtly angular or rounded, a complementary shape should be chosen. For example, if a client has a sharply angular face frame, a rounded brow shape will soften the sharp lines (Figure 7–4). Conversely, if a client has an overly round face, an arched brow shape will bring dimension and harmony to her face (Figure 7–5). Eyebrow expert, Damone Roberts, agrees. "Eyebrows should complement the face. If you have a round face, the last thing you want is round brows. Similarly, a rounder brow softens the lines of an angular face."

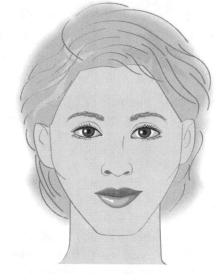

Figure 7–4.   Angular facial frame is balanced with rounded brow shape

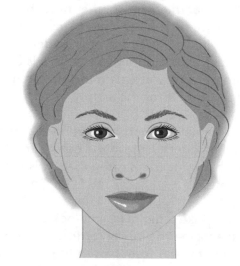

Figure 7–5.   A rounded facial frame is balanced with angular brows

Oftentimes, a client's facial frame is neither predominantly angled nor rounded. When this is the case, you and your client can choose an angled, rounded, or softly angled brow shape. If the client would like to see the impact of an angled versus a rounded brow, you can try both, one over each eye (Figure 7–6). The more appealing shape is easy to choose when you see the options side by side. The appropriate beginning and ending points must be maintained for this visual test to be effective.

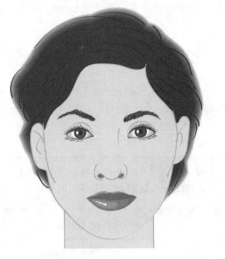

Figure 7–6. One side has a rounded brow; the other side has a more angular shape

The Eyebrow Length

The eyebrow length is the horizontal measurement from Point A to Point B, where Point A = the be-

ginning point and Point B = the ending point (Figure 7–7). Measuring for eyebrow length is a three-dimensional measurement. The correct length is an extremely important facet of eyebrow shape selection. If the length is wrong, the eyebrow will look wrong and the entire face will look out of balance.

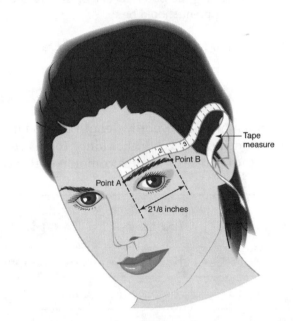

Figure 7–7. Measure horizontally from Point A to Point B to obtain the correct length of the eyebrow. Point A = the beginning point and Point B = the ending point. This is a three dimensional measurement and must be done with a tape measure, instead of a flat ruler.

Practice Sheet for Measuring for the Ideal Length for the Eyebrow.

Step #1: Locate your ideal beginning point, Point A, by taking a ruler and holding it vertically upward from the inner corner of the eye. If there is no hair at that location, use an eyebrow pencil to place a dot there.

Step #2: Locate your ideal ending point, Point B, by taking a ruler and holding it at the base of the nose, at a diagonal angle, intersecting the outer corner of the eye and beyond. If there is no brow hair there, place a dot at the place where the ending point should be.

Step #3: Using a soft tape measure, measure horizontally from Point A to Point B. Record the optimal length for your eyebrow. _____

Most women have an eyebrow length that is between $1^7/8$ inches and $2^3/8$ inches long. There are exceptions, of course. The most common eyebrow length is $2^1/8$ inches. Refer to Table 7–1 for samples of eyebrow shapes for each of the most common lengths.

TABLE 7–1.   THE MOST COMMON EYEBROW LENGTHS

Eyebrow Length	Measured Length	Eyebrow Shape
$1^7/8$ inches	_____	
2 inches	_____	
$2^1/8$ inches	_____	
$2^3/8$ inches	_____	

Open or Closed Ending Point

Choosing whether the ending point of the eyebrow will be open, closed, or below-closed depends on whether the face requires the illusion of lengthening, such as in the case of a round face.

If the ending point is open (Figure 7–8), it is above an imaginary horizontal line, which is drawn from the beginning point outward. Choosing an eyebrow shape that has an open ending point will provide the illusion of lengthening the middle and lower zones of the face, and thus the entire face. It will also draw the focus upward and appear to provide lift in the upper zone. A person with a round face will benefit from having an open ending point.

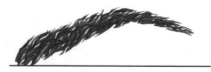

Figure 7–8.   Eyebrow with open ending point

If the ending point is closed (Figure 7–9), it touches the imaginary horizontal line. It does not create an illusionary change unless the brow is flat (unarched). Most eyebrow shapes have a closed ending point.

Figure 7–9.   Eyebrow with closed ending point

If you are enhancing an eyebrow, you cannot achieve a desired illusionary change by designing an eyebrow shape that has a below-closed ending point (Figure 7–10) because it tends to draw the eye downward. A below-closed eyebrow goes below the imaginary horizontal line. This type of eyebrow is seen most often on Oriental women, but can be found on women of any nationality. You may consider changing a below-closed eyebrow to one that ends at or above the line. On rare occasions, if a large enough portion of the brow goes below the line, you may have no alternative but to maintain a below-closed ending point, enhancing the brow where possible.

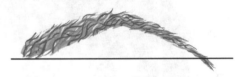

Figure 7–10.   Eyebrow with below-closed ending point

Practice Worksheet 1

Correct the beginning point of the eyebrow by sketching in additional brow hairs.

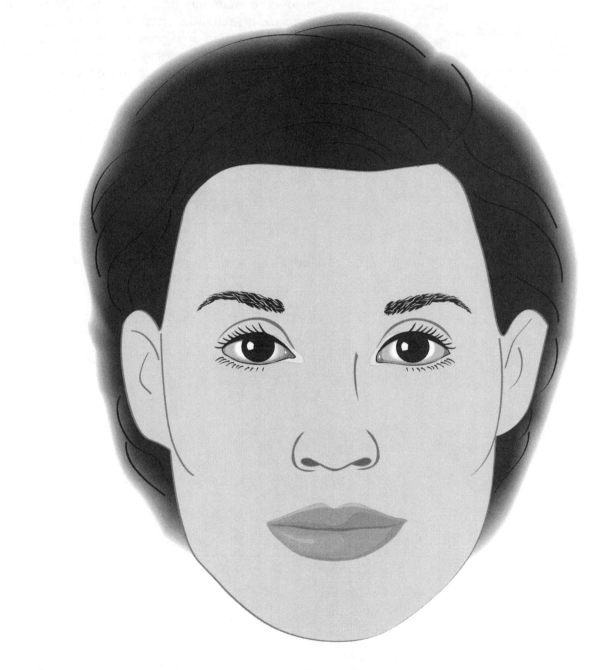

Figure 7–11.   Worksheet—Correct the beginning point by drawing in or whiting out brow hairs.

Practice Worksheet 2

Alter the ending point so the brow stops at the correct place.

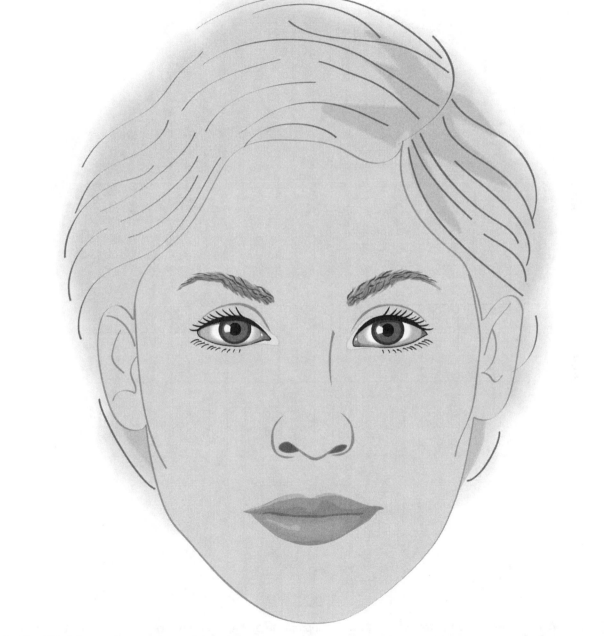

Figure 7–12. Worksheet—Correct the ending point.

Practice Worksheet 3

Sketch a well-balanced eyebrow using the six brow element guidelines.

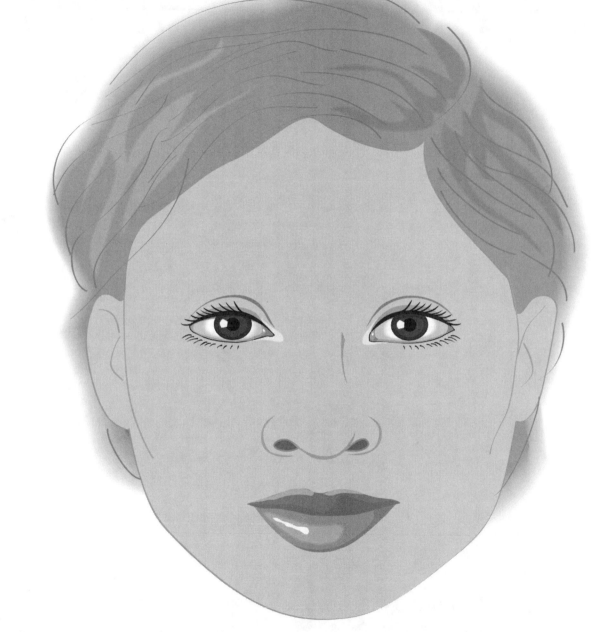

Figure 7–13.   Worksheet—Identify the face shape. Draw an appropriate eyebrow for this face. Make sure the beginning and ending points are correct.

REFERENCES

D'Angelo, J., Lees, M., Dean, P. S., Miller, E., Dietz, S., Zani, A., & Hinds, C. 2003. *Milady's standard comprehensive training for estheticians.* Clifton Park, NY: Delmar Learning.

James, J. (2002, March). Chalk it up to the Boho revival: Anorexic arches are out and natural brows are back: Here are four ways to get yours in shape. *Teen People*, 149.

Villa, L. P. (1987). *Cosmetology: The art of making up.* Toronto, Canada: Gage Educational Publishing Company.

Chapter 8

CORRECTIVE TECHNIQUES TO THE EYEBROW TO ENHANCE THE FEATURES OF THE FACE

Learning Objectives

After reading this chapter, you should be able to:

1. Describe the corrective technique to the eyebrow that can make the eyes look less wide set.

2. Explain how to make close-set eyes appear more balanced through a corrective technique to the eyebrow.

3. List the two attributes of the eyebrow arch that can be changed to create a cosmetic illusion to enhance the features of the face.

4. Specify the illusion that is created by selecting an eyebrow shape that has very little arch.

5. Discuss the effect on the face, either lengthening or widening, of having a highly sloped eyebrow with an open ending point.

6. Identify the point along the eyebrow before which the arch should never be placed.

Utilizing corrective techniques to the eyebrows entails modifying an eyebrow to cosmetically enhance imperfections in the client's features. Such imperfections can include eyes that are close set, a nose that has a wide base, lips that are narrow, and a wide upper zone, among others. As you begin to perform eyebrow makeovers, it will appear that there is an overabundant number of considerations in the process of "eyebrow design." As you work with each client, you will learn to prioritize the most important issues and find solutions where possible.

You may come across a client with incongruous features such that enhancing one feature may work in opposition to the solution of another feature. For example, you may have a client who has a long face, wide-set eyes, and large facial features (eyes, nose, and lips). During your analysis, you may decide to choose:

- a thick brow shape to be consistent with the large features
- a brow with very little arch to create the illusion of added width to the upper zone
- to move the brow inward to make the eyes appear less wide set

However, an eyebrow that is relatively flat tends to emphasize a large nose, and moving the eyebrow inward on a narrow face will tend to make it appear narrower. The point is that you will not be able to cure all beauty issues with an eyebrow alteration. However, if you focus on the most important ones and perform the techniques that will enhance them, it will go a long way toward enhancing the client's overall appearance.

Let us now revisit the 10 facial features outlined in Chapter 5. We will discuss how to make corrective technique changes to the eyebrows to improve those features.

Corrective Techniques to Improve Eye Set

The beginning point of the eyebrow can be moved inward or outward to give the illusion of changing an undesired eye set. If the eyes are wide set (Figure 8–1), the beginning point can be moved inward by powdering or penciling in at the beginning point.

This gives the illusion of a less wide-set look (Figure 8–2). Recall that lip width and nose width should be considered when deciding whether or not to make this correction. If the lips are proportionately balanced with the eyes, meaning both the eyes and the lips are wide set, then you may choose not to move the beginning point inward. Conversely, you are more likely to move the beginning point inward if the lips are narrow and the eyes are wide set.

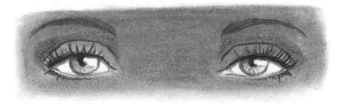

Figure 8–1.   Before—Wide-set eyes

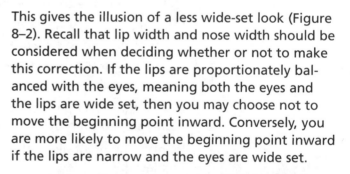

Figure 8–2.   After—Adding fill-in to the beginning point makes the eyes appear less wide set.

If a client's eyes are close set (Figure 8–3), then the opposite cosmetic correction can be made. Move the beginning point of the eyebrow outward by removing brow hair at the inner corners of the existing eyebrow. Do not remove too many eyebrow hairs at the beginning point.

When this correction is done carefully (Figure 8–4), the eyebrow will begin ever so slightly outside the inner corner of the eye and give the illusion that the eyes are not so close set. As mentioned in previous chapters, do not make the mistake of aligning the new beginning point with the base of the nose, as this will render the features out of proportion.

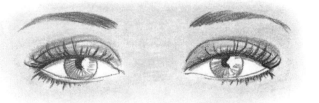

Figure 8–3.   Before—Close-set eyes

Figure 8–4.   After—Removing just a few brow hairs at the beginning point makes the eyes look less close set.

Corrective Techniques to Improve Eye Size and Eye Orientation

When considering eye size, the key strategy is to be consistent with the eyes. This will provide balance and not draw attention to an undesired eye size. If a person has small eyes, she should not choose a thick and dramatic eyebrow shape (Figure 8–5). The client's features will be more harmonious and balanced if a thin to medium shape is chosen (Figure 8–6).

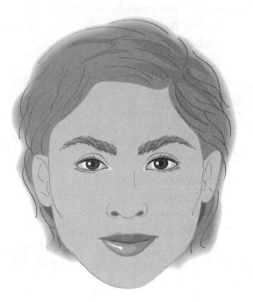

Figure 8–5.   Wrong—Thick eyebrows and small eyes make this face look disproportionate.

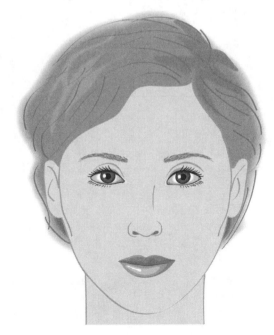

Figure 8–6.   Right—Small eyes and a thin eyebrow makes the face harmonious and balanced.

Likewise, if a person has large eyes, the brow thickness choice should not be a thin eyebrow shape (Figure 8–7). Rather, it is best to crown them with a medium to thick eyebrow, especially if the client's other features are medium to large (Figure 8–8).

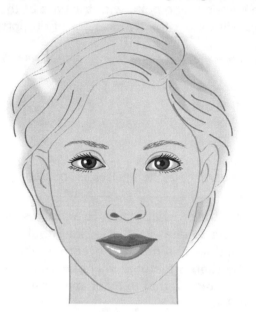

Figure 8–7.   Wrong—Thin eyebrows and large eyes make the face look inconsistent.

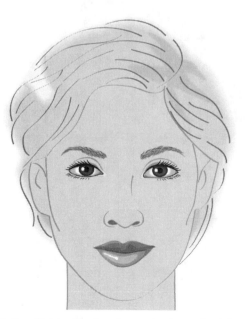

Figure 8–8.   Right—Medium/large-sized eyes look best with medium/large-sized eyebrows.

When considering eye orientation, the strategy is to work opposite the undesired characteristic. Recall from Chapter 5 the three types of eye orientation. The ideal orientation for the eyes is the almond shape where the eye ends slightly upward (Figure 8–9). There is no correction necessary for this eye shape.

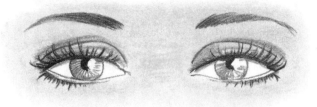

Figure 8–9.   The almond-shaped eye is the ideal shape.

The even-shaped eye (Figure 8–10) is a common orientation for the eye and does not require a correction unless the client would like her eyes to appear more almond-like. The drooping eye (Figure 8–11) can be made to look more like the almond eye by choosing an eyebrow shape that ends opposite the eye's ending point direction (Figure 8–12). For example, if a woman has drooping eyes that end downward, her new brow shape should have an open ending point. This will draw the attention upward and balance the drooping eye.

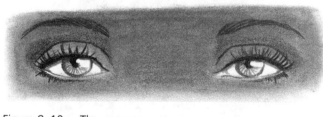

Figure 8–10.   The even eye

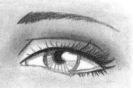
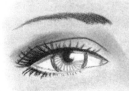

Figure 8–11.   The drooping eye

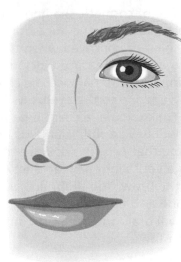

Figure 8–12.   Corrective technique for a drooping eye. Make sure the new eyebrow shape has an open ending point.

Corrective Techniques to Improve the Appearance of the Nose

The characteristics of the nose can be cosmetically improved by making changes to the eyebrows. Shading is the simplest and most effective corrective technique to improve a large nose. However, if you wish to further improve the size of the nose by changing the eyebrow, the following changes can be made.

1. Make sure the brow length is fully extended to the correct ending point. When a person has only the first half or two-thirds of the eyebrow and it is not extended to its correct ending point, the attention will focus on the nose (Figure 8–13). Conversely, when the brow is the correct length, the focus will be more toward the eyes (Figure 8–14).
2. Avoid a flat (unarched) eyebrow shape. A flat eyebrow, while it has other corrective influences, will also create an inward focus toward the nose. An upward sloping eyebrow turns the focus away from the nose.

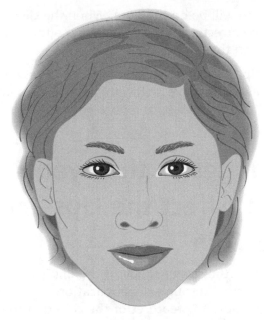

Figure 8–13.   An eyebrow that does not extend to its correct ending point will cause the focus to be on the nose.

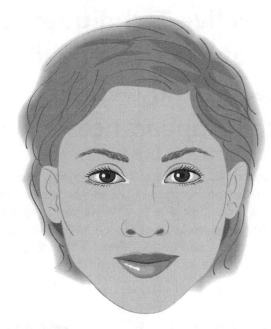

Figure 8–14.   After the eyebrow is extended to the correct length, the focus is on the beautiful eyes.

3. Change from a thick shape to a medium-width shape. This is a tricky correction because if the eyebrow is either too thick or too thin, the

focus will be on the nose. When the client has the correct eyebrow thickness, the focus will be on the eyes.

If the tip of the nose is ball-shaped, an eyebrow that has a distinctive arch will take the focus away from the roundness of the nose and pull it up to the eyes.

Changes to the Eyebrows that Affect the Lips and the Chin

Improving the size or shape of the lips is optimally accomplished through the application of lip liner and lip color. Any features of the chin that the client wishes to change will best be improved through the use of cosmetic shading and contouring techniques. However, the appearance of the lips and the chin are improved when they are in proportion to all other features, including the eyebrows. It is important to balance the chin and the lips in the lower zone to the eyebrows in the upper zone. For example, a client who has a pear-shaped face will have a full, rounded chin. The eyebrow shape that provides balance to her chin is one that has a very slight arch at the two-thirds point along the brow. The slight arch will widen her upper zone and the arch placed at the two-thirds point will draw the attention outward, further widening the upper zone.

The features of the eyebrow shape you select can provide balance to the lips and the chin. By providing balance among the zones, you are enhancing the client's overall attractiveness.

Corrective Techniques to Improve the Forehead Breadth and Overall Facial Appearance

If the forehead is found to be undesirably prominent or the hairline shape is wide, the upper zone of the face can be made to look narrower by manipulating two features of the arch. The two parts of the arch that can be changed are the height of the arch and the location of the arch.

The height of the arch varies from flat to highly arched. Figures 8–15 through 8–18 show four eyebrow shapes with the same length, thickness, and arch location. The arch location is at the two-thirds point on each brow. The only difference between the brows is the amount of height of the arch.

The eyebrow shapes that are mostly flat (Figure 8–15) and slightly arched (Figure 8–16) will create the illusion of having a wider upper zone. Use a flat eyebrow shape if your client has a forehead she believes is too narrow. The flat eyebrow shape will provide the illusion of width so the face will not appear as long.

The eyebrows that have the medium arch (Figure 8–17) and the highest arch (Figure 8–18) will give

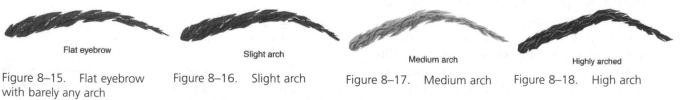

Flat eyebrow

Slight arch

Medium arch

Highly arched

Figure 8–15.   Flat eyebrow with barely any arch

Figure 8–16.   Slight arch

Figure 8–17.   Medium arch

Figure 8–18.   High arch

All eyebrows are exactly the same EXCEPT for arch height.

the illusion of lengthening the face. That is because a brow shape with a higher arch has a greater slope. A greater slope will lengthen the lower two zones and create the illusion of lengthening the entire face. Therefore, choose an eyebrow shape with a high arch if a client has either a wide forehead and/or a round face shape.

The location of the arch can also create an illusion of narrowness or width in the upper zone, and hence in the overall facial appearance. Figures 8–19 through 8–22 show an eyebrow shape with the same length, thickness, and arch height. The only difference between the four eyebrows is the location of the arch; that is, at what point along the brow the arch is placed.

Figure 8–19 shows the arch at the half-way point along the brow. Choosing a shape with an arch location at that point will serve to narrow the upper zone, and hence the overall facial appearance. Choose this arch location if the forehead tends to be wide. Do not create an eyebrow shape in which the arch is closer in than the half-way point. This eyebrow will look unnatural and will cause the focus to be on the ill-conceived brow instead of the client's beautiful eyes.

Figure 8–22 shows an eyebrow with the arch at the two-thirds point. This location of the arch will serve to widen the upper zone. Choose this arch location if the client has a narrow forehead.

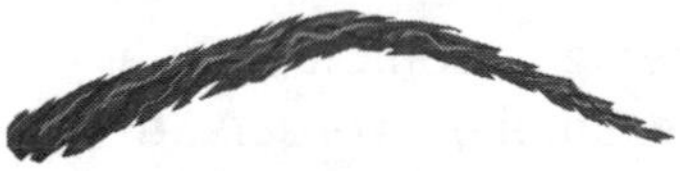

Arch at mid-point of brow

Figure 8–19.   Arch at ½ point along the brow

Arch slightly beyond mid-point of brow

Figure 8–20.   Arch slightly beyond the ½ point

Arch at two-thirds location on the brow

Figure 8–21.   Arch at the ⅔ point along the brow

Arch is located beyond the two-thirds point on the brow

Figure 8–22.   Arch slightly beyond the ⅔ point

All eyebrows are exactly the same EXCEPT for the location of the arch.

Hairstyle with Respect to Corrective Techniques to the Eyebrow

The key to optimizing the relationship between hairstyle and eyebrows is to focus on ideal brow thickness and color.

While there are no rules or standards that dictate eyebrow thickness for different hairstyles, common sense and esthetic judgment will assist you in maintaining a balance between the two. For example, if a woman consistently wears her hair pulled back, she may be inclined to pare down her brow thickness. On the other hand, if a woman's hairstyle is long, thick, and wavy, she may be inclined to wear a thicker shape.

The color choice for the eyebrow is greatly impacted by the color choice of the hair, and the same is true for the other way around. Choosing an eyebrow fill-in color that complements the hair color will enhance a person's overall appearance. Focusing on an esthetically pleasing thickness and color provides a correction and improvement to the overall appearance.

Corrective Techniques to the Eyebrow to Counter the Effects of Age

Each time you design an esthetically pleasing eyebrow for an older client, you are performing corrective techniques that counter the effects of aging (Figure 8–23). This occurs in three ways.

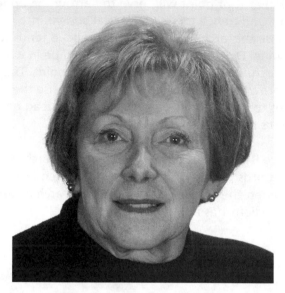

Figure 8–23. Before—A mature client before an eyebrow makeover.

1. Selecting a shape that adds arch to the existing eyebrow and/or one that has an open ending point provides an instant nonsurgical eyelift (Figure 8–24).

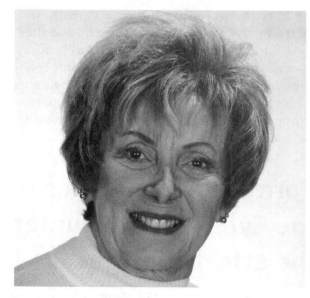

Figure 8–24. After—After the eyebrow enhancement, the client's eyes are dramatically lifted.

2. Filling in the outer part of the eyebrow makes the older client appear younger. This is because older women very often do not have brow hairs on the outer third of their eyebrow whereas younger women do.
3. Choosing an eyebrow powder for fill-in allows you to cover brow hairs that have grayed over time. Adding taupes and browns to a graying eyebrow will transform the aging brow into a more youthful looking one.

Changes to the Eyebrow that Can Affect Overall Style

The brow shape should serve to complement a client's overall style. For example, a conservative person who wishes to appear consistent with that image can choose an eyebrow shape that is thin to medium, that gently arches at the two-thirds point, and tapers off to a closed ending point.

The late Kevyn Aucoin recognized that the eyebrows could be used to create or sustain certain images. In his book *Making Faces*, he wrote, ". . . while some may hesitate and balk at the idea of changing one's brow shape, one only needs to think of Marlene Dietrich, Elizabeth Taylor, Audrey Hepburn or Diana Ross to realize how altering the shape can help create a signature look." The shapes he used included styles such as seductive, unkempt, waifish, youthful, and tomboyish. Table 8–1 shows examples of eyebrow shapes that are consistent with each of the seven personality types introduced in Chapter 5.

Selecting an eyebrow shape can actually be fun, especially if you have a client who likes to experiment. Be sure to maintain the beginning point, ending point, and correct length for the client. Then, if the brow shape works with her style and taste, let the imagination fly and enjoy!

TABLE 8–1. EYEBROW SHAPES CONSISTENT WITH PERSONALITY TYPES

Personality Type	Example Eyebrow Shape for Each Personality Type
Natural	
Conservative	
Artistic	
Extravagant	
Relaxed/Carefree	
Intense	
Demure	

REFERENCES

Aucoin, K. (1997). *Making faces.* New York: Little Brown and Company.

D'Angelo, J., Lees, M., Dean, P. S., Miller, E., Dietz, S., Zani, A., & Hinds, C. 2003. *Milady's standard comprehensive training for estheticians.* Clifton Park, NY: Delmar Learning.

Chapter 9

EYEBROW DESIGN METHODS

Learning Objectives

After reading this chapter, you should be able to:

1. Identify two methods of "eyebrow design."

2. List the advantages and disadvantages of designing eyebrows via the free-hand method.

3. Describe the advantages and disadvantages of using additional shaping tools for the process of "eyebrow design."

4. Describe the distinction between brow enhancement and total eyebrow creation.

Two Methods Used to Design the Eyebrows

The process of "eyebrow design" can be performed using either the freehand method or the template/strip method. The freehand method involves utilizing rules and esthetic judgment, along with brow powders or pencils, to design an attractive eyebrow for your client. The template/strip method encompasses all the elements used for the freehand method, plus adds templates or strips to assist the designer. The templates or strips, sometimes called "stencils," contain an eyebrow shape that is used as a fill-in or hair removal guide.

Your choice of one method over the other depends on your priorities while you are performing eyebrow enhancement, and the technical abilities and esthetic talents you possess. When you perform eyebrow enhancement on a client, your first priority may be quickness and efficiency. If that is the case, you may be inclined to work freehand. If your top priority is providing the client with a high degree of symmetry and pinpoint accuracy, you may opt to use the additional tools to assist you.

If you are artistically inclined and perform much of your work using the esthetic, right side of your brain, freehand eyebrow enhancement may be your best option. On the other hand, if you are most comfortable working with the technical, left side of your brain, you may best perform this service using templates and strips in your eyebrow enhancement work.

These generalizations provide a guideline to help you choose the best method for you. However, since most professionals' priorities vary for each client, and most professionals work from both sides of the brain, it is in your best interest to be able to perform both methods of eyebrow enhancement, sometimes simultaneously and sometimes individually. To determine which method to use under different circumstances, refer to Table 9–1, which outlines the advantages and disadvantages of each method.

TABLE 9–1.   ADVANTAGES AND DISADVANTAGES OF THE TWO METHODS OF EYEBROW ENHANCEMENT

	Freehand	Templates and Other Tools
Advantages	1. You can work relatively quickly and efficiently. 2. Each pair of eyebrows will be unique, although you will repeat certain shapes as you find those that are the most common ones. 3. You will require fewer tools than when using the template method.	1. You can enhance an eyebrow so that it will be perfectly symmetrical. 2. You can repeat the exact same, beautiful eyebrow over and over again for the same client. With the freehand method, the eyebrow is likely to look different each time it is enhanced. 3. The clients will be able to purchase some of the tools to enable them to fill in their brows at home. Using the templates, they will be able to attain symmetry. If they perform the fill-in function using the freehand method, they may be unable to make their eyebrows even.

(continues)

	Freehand	Templates and Other Tools
Disadvantages	1. Attaining absolute symmetry is not possible.	1. Learning to use templates or other tools may take extra time. However, once the client's shape is selected, the template method may prove to be quicker because the professional can use the selected shape each time the client comes in for hair removal.
	2. It takes time, practice, and natural artistic talent that some professionals do not possess. People who are more technically oriented may have an easier time working with tools.	2. The beauty professional will require additional tools over and above those used by a professional using the freehand method.
	3. Results can be unpredictable. The client may like the outcome of a brow makeover, but the beauty professional may have difficulty duplicating the result. When a person is having an "off" day, working freehand may produce unwanted results.	3. It takes time and effort to purchase the additional tools.

Two Different Approaches to Eyebrow Enhancement

There are two different approaches to "eyebrow design:" brow enhancement and total brow creation. The approach is not a choice but instead, is based on the existing condition of the client's eyebrows.

Brow enhancement is the process of designing a pair of eyebrows using the rules of proper eyebrow placement and subjective esthetic input, in conjunction with the existing eyebrow shape and arch as guidelines. Brow enhancement is performed when the client has enough existing eyebrow hairs so the professional can clearly see the natural line of the eyebrow and its arch.

After identifying the ideal beginning and ending points, the existing eyebrow can be added to or subtracted from to bring about the desired result. Working with the existing eyebrow will create less upkeep for the client in the way of hair removal and fill-in.

Total brow creation is the process of designing a pair of eyebrows by creating an entirely new eyebrow shape based on the rules of proper eyebrow placement and subjective esthetic input. You will need to work from this approach if the client has a few or no existing brow hairs with which to work.

Examples of when you will perform total eyebrow creation are:

- when someone has eyebrows that are so light they are not visible
- during a makeover on a client who desires a high fashion eyebrow; you may be called on to cover the existing brow and create a whole new eyebrow
- in the case of a client who has undergone chemotherapy and/or radiation, and has lost eyebrow hair as a result
- where a client has experienced hair loss due to an illness such as alopecia
- when a person has removed too many brow hairs that have never grown back

When you are performing total eyebrow creation, it is helpful to have certain shapes in mind for each different face shape you may encounter. Table 9–2 shows suggested eyebrow shapes for each face shape. This will help you with the difficult task of creating an entirely new eyebrow shape for your client.

TABLE 9–2.   SUGGESTED EYEBROW SHAPES FOR EACH FACE SHAPE

Face Shape	Optimal Eyebrow Shape	Description of the Brow Shape
Oval		The arch can be anywhere between the $1/2$ to $2/3$ point on the brow. A closed ending point is best. A classic eyebrow shape, neither sharply angled nor totally rounded.
Long		The arch should be minimal and closer to the $2/3$ point. Closed ending point; a flat eyebrow shape will create the desired illusion of widening the face.
Square		The arch can either be at the $1/2$ point or the $2/3$ point, depending on location of jawline (which is based on narrowness or width of face). Closed ending point; a well-arched eyebrow shape will balance the jawline of the square shaped face. If very sharp, straight lines characterize the jawline, use a similar brow shape as suggested above, except with a softened arch.
Round		The arch needs to be in between the $1/2$ to the $2/3$ point on the brow, closer to the $1/2$ point. This will provide the illusion of narrowing the upper zone. An open ending point will draw the attention upward and give the illusion of elongating the lower zones of the rounded face.

(continues)

Face Shape	Optimal Eyebrow Shape	Description of the Brow Shape
Inverted Triangle or Heart		If the client's hairstyle causes the triangular face shape to look like an oval, then refer to suggestions for the oval face shape. If hairstyle does not hide the wide forehead of the client and you wish to conceal it, choose a shape whose arch is close to the $1/2$ point. This will create an illusion of narrowing the upper zone. An open ending point would be optimal, but a closed ending point can be used, especially if client's hairstyle makes the face look more oval.
Diamond		The arch should be closer to the $2/3$ point to widen the upper zone. The ending point is best if it is closed and the brow shape barely arched. This will serve to create the illusion of widening the upper zone so it is similar to the upper zone of an oval face. In addition, a diamond-shaped face is usually long. Wearing a brow shape with a low degree of arch will make the face appear less long.
Pear		The arch is optimally placed closer to the $2/3$ point on the brow, which gives the illusion of widening the upper zone. On a face with a narrow upper zone, the recommendation for the ending point would normally be to keep it closed to further provide this illusion of widening that narrow upper zone. In the case of a pear-shaped face, however, it is beneficial to open the ending point in order to draw the focus away from the full chin.
Hexagon		Since an oval and a hexagon face have similar measurements, one can use a similar brow shape for both face types. However, a softer, more rounded eyebrow may soften the angles of the hexagon-shaped face.

Chapter 10

PERFORMING EYEBROW DESIGN AND ENHANCEMENT

Learning Objectives

After reading this chapter, you should be able to:

1. Describe the importance of the client consultation and how it will save the professional time in the long run.

2. List the three pieces of information you will learn about the client from the eyebrow enhancement questionnaire.

3. Demonstrate how to fill out a client profile for eyebrow enhancement services.

4. Describe the benefits of using the eyebrow prescription form and demonstrate how to complete it.

5. Perform an eyebrow enhancement service using the template method.

6. Perform an eyebrow enhancement makeover using the freehand method.

7. List the benefits of knowing how to use both methods in performing an eyebrow makeover.

Tools you will need:

- ruler
- pen or pencil (pencil is preferable)
- a "white out" product
- tape measure to measure eyebrow length

The Importance of the Client Consultation

Performing the client consultation is an essential first step in giving your clients the best results from any service you provide, including their eyebrow makeover. In order to provide an effective consultation, you must:

- listen well to learn what the client wants
- earn client trust by responding appropriately and speaking diplomatically regarding sensitive issues
- communicate effectively to introduce the client to new methods, techniques, and products
- gather all of the necessary information about the client to provide the service safely, correctly, and to the highest degree of satisfaction

It is simply not enough to seat clients and begin doing what you think will best improve their appearance. Today's women are more educated and discerning with regard to their tastes and desires. It is up to you to maintain a dialogue with your client so that you can match what she wants to what is esthetically appropriate. At the same time, today's women are entirely too busy to know all that you know with regard to the latest techniques and products that will benefit them. They are counting on you to share that information.

An effective "eyebrow design" consultation should take between 10 and 30 minutes, depending on your speed and experience. Each subsequent time the client comes in for hair removal, all you need to do is pull out her previously recorded consultation forms and update them for any health, medication, or preference changes. You will be completely ready to work.

Consultation Forms

There are three recommended forms for use during the client consultation. The first form is an eyebrow enhancement questionnaire (Figure 10–1). The client completes this form as she arrives for her first eyebrow consultation. It should be updated as changes in her health and medication habits occur. This questionnaire provides the beauty professional with information about the client's likes and dislikes about her eyebrows, preferred hair removal method(s), and health condition and medications. The professional fills out the second form, the client profile (Figure 10–2), during the consultation. After the assessments are made and recorded on the client profile, the professional will have the information needed to design the client's eyebrows. Last, the eyebrow prescription form (Figure 10–3) is a checklist of the products used during the eyebrow makeover that the client may wish to purchase for home use.

The consultation forms should be filled out regardless of which method of eyebrow design you choose. This is because both methods depend on a clear assessment of the client's facial features and eyebrows, which are performed to attain the best result.

EYEBROW ENHANCEMENT QUESTIONNAIRE

Client Name: _____ Date: _____

A. Your Eyebrows

    1. What do you like about your eyebrows?

    _____

    _____

    2. What would you like to change about your eyebrows?

    _____

    _____

B. Your Health and Medications

    3. Have you used Accutane in the last seven years? _____

    4. Are you currently using Accutane?_____

    5. Are you currently using Retin-A?_____ Renova?_____

    6. Are you currently taking blood thinners such as Coumadin?_____

    7. Do you use any of the following: Salicyclic acid, alphahydroxy acids, enzymes, scrubs, depilatory creams, vitamin C creams? If so, please list and describe your frequency of use.

    _____

    _____

    8. Do you have: ❑ Diabetes ❑ Cancer ❑ High Blood Pressure ❑ Acne
                   ❑ Phlebitis ❑ Autoimmune Diseases such as Lupus ❑ Sunburn

    9. Have you ever had an adverse reaction after hair removal? If yes, specify the type of hair removal and the adverse reaction you had.

    _____

    _____

    10. Have you been in the sun or in a tanning bed within the last 48 hours? _____

C. Your Preferred Method of Hair Removal

    11. What type of hair removal do you wish to have done today? _____

I have answered all of the questions to the best of my knowledge. I understand that the professional may refuse to provide epilation services because of certain health conditions and that it is in my best interest if the service is not provided. I also understand that there may be swelling or irritation in the areas that are waxed or otherwise epilated. This is only a temporary condition.

Client's Signature _____ Date_____

Figure 10–1. Eyebrow Enhancement Questionnaire

CLIENT PROFILE FOR EYEBROW ENHANCEMENT SERVICES

Name: _____ Date: _____

1. Face Shape: ❑ Round ❑ Long ❑ Square ❑ Oval ❑ Inverted Triangle or Heart ❑ Pear
    ❑ Diamond ❑ Hexagon
2. Circle zone(s) that is/are wide.   Upper   Middle   Lower
3. Circle zone(s) that is/are long.   Upper   Middle   Lower
4. Indicate client's eye set.   Close   Well   Wide
5. Overall size of features: Small   Medium   Large
6. Size of nose _____
7. Is lip width proportionate to eye width? ❑ yes   ❑ no
8. Eye orientation: Almond   Even   Drooping
9. Color tone: Warm   Cool
10. Personality type: ❑ Natural ❑ Conservative ❑ Artistic ❑ Extravagant
    ❑ Relaxed/carefree ❑ Intense ❑ Demure ❑ Other_____
11. Age group: ❑ Twenties ❑ Thirties ❑ Forties ❑ Fifties ❑ Sixties or older
12. Type of work _____
13. Current condition of eyebrows:

    _____

    _____

14. What features would the client like to cosmetically enhance?

    _____

    _____

15. Ideal length of eyebrow: ❑ 1⁷/₈" ❑ 2" ❑ 2¹/₈" ❑ 2³/₈" ❑ Other
16. Other important information:

    _____

    _____

Figure 10–2.   Client Profile

EYEBROW PRESCRIPTION FORM

In order to maintain beautiful, symmetrical eyebrows, the following items are recommended:

❑ Eyebrow brush/comb

❑ Tweezers

❑ Brow setting product

❑ Eyebrow powder in _____ colors

❑ Eyebrow pencil in _____ colors

❑ Eyebrow powder applicator

❑ Template in _____ shape

❑ Brow perfecting strips in _____ shape

❑ It is recommended that the client have _____ (type of hair removal) performed every _____ weeks.

You can schedule your next appointment before leaving today. We will call you to confirm.

(Your Salon Name)

(Salon Telephone Number)

Figure 10–3.   Eyebrow Prescription Form

The Template/ Strip Method

Introduction

The template/strip method will assist the professional in selecting an attractive and well-suited eyebrow shape for the client. This method guarantees the highest degree of symmetry when performed correctly. The professional can teach clients how to fill in their eyebrows evenly, and clients can purchase the templates and/or strips in order to perform symmetrical fill-in at home.

Room Setup

1. Make sure the service area is clean and orderly.
2. Have a disposable neck wrap and client cape handy.
3. Place the client profile and the eyebrow prescription form on a clipboard near the treatment area.
4. Have all necessary tools presanitized and all supplies ready to use.

Tools and Supplies

- ruler or other flat-edged device
- cotton pads
- nonoily, fragrance-free eye makeup remover
- eyebrow powders
- spatula to remove brow powder from compact
- clean tray or dish for powders
- disposable applicators
- eyebrow brush/comb
- Q-tips
- cotton balls
- alcohol
- tissues
- eyebrow pencils
- brow setting product;
- nippers or manicure scissors
- templates and/or brow perfecting strips in a variety of shapes and sizes
- large handheld mirror
- sanitizing solution and container
- sanitized tweezers
- equipment and supplies for other desired hair removal methods

Client Preparation

The client will complete the eyebrow enhancement questionnaire on arrival. Give the client a few moments to complete the form. Greet the client and take the questionnaire. Escort the client to the treatment room or area. Seat the client while glancing over her answers and information. Secure a disposable neck wrap and drape the client with a makeup cape. Pull the hair away from the face either by using a turban, towel, or Velcro™ headband. Assess the client's appearance while making notes on her client profile. Wash or sanitize your hands in the presence of your client.

Consider the condition of the client's eyebrow. Perform brow enhancement if there are enough existing hairs to see the natural line of the eyebrow and to distinguish the arch. Begin at Step 1 and work through all of the steps. Perform total eyebrow creation if there are few or no existing hairs. Begin at Step 1 and work through only the steps that are applicable.

Step-by-Step Procedure Using the Template/Strip Method for Brow Enhancement

The following procedure will be performed using both the client's existing brow shape and templates/strips as the guides for the eyebrow design of this client (Figure 10–4).

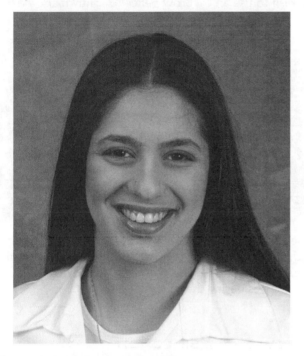

Figure 10–4   Before brow enhancement

Note: We recommend that the client sit upright for the consultation/design and lay slightly reclined for the hair removal service. Each professional can choose how to position the client based on the client and the practitioner's comfort and ease.

1. Remove eyebrow makeup using eye makeup remover and a cotton pad.

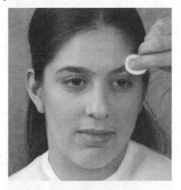

2. Identify the client's eye set and note the client's lip length relative to eye width.

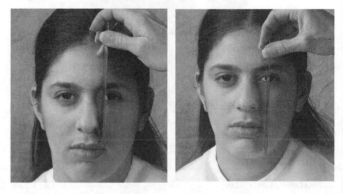

3. Brush the eyebrows upward and outward. Trim long eyebrow hairs, if necessary. Locate and study the arch and the natural line of the eyebrow.

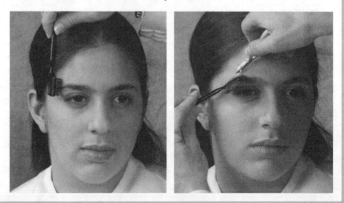

4. If the client has tuft hair, give her a handheld mirror to show her how those hairs look. Discuss the possible removal of tuft hairs that are outside the body of the brow and show her how she will look if she chooses to have them removed. Study the length and amount of all of the excess hair, including the tuft hair, and decide on an appropriate hair removal method that will be performed after the eyebrow is designed.

5. Touch the eyebrows to discern the texture of the hairs. Decide whether the client will benefit from using a brow setting product. Also, decide on brow fill-in color choices as you study the coloring of the client's hair and brows.

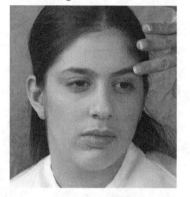

6. Using a ruler or measuring device, locate the optimal beginning and ending points for the brow. Measure to find the optimal brow length using a nonstiff tape measure. (If you are performing total eyebrow creation, you may wish to use an eyebrow pencil to lightly mark the beginning and ending points.)

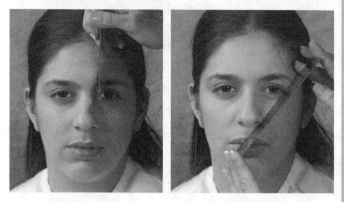

7. Select one or more templates that have the desired length and thickness. Table 10–1 lists the choices you will make, and the features you will need to study to make these choices during the shape selection process.

TABLE 10–1. CHOICES FOR EYEBROW SHAPE SELECTION

Choose/Decide	By Studying This Feature
Optimal eyebrow thickness	Overall feature size
Brow shape, either rounded or angular	The lines of the frame of the face
Arch location	The width of the upper zone
Arch height	The width of the upper zone and the length of the face
Ending point, open or closed	The face shape and/or the length and width of the facial zones; also the eye orientation
A complementary shape for the client	Overall style and personality (hair, clothing, and work)
Whether the beginning point should be moved inward or outward	The client's eye set
Corrective techniques to perform on the eyebrows	Those specific features the client wishes to improve

Use the arch and the natural line of the eyebrow in conjunction with the choices outlined in Table 10–1 to select the ideal shape. The arch on the template should match closely to the existing arch of the eyebrow, even if there are sparse hairs in that area. It is paramount that the correct ending point location is part of the newly selected shape.

If you are performing total eyebrow creation, you must consider many factors in selecting an appealing eyebrow shape for the client. First, ask the client how her brows looked before she lost her brow hair. Ask her what she liked and did not like about them. Next, consider her overall feature size to make sure the shape you choose is consistent with her feature size. Finally, take into consideration the client's face shape when selecting a brow shape for her. Use the information provided in Table 9–2, Suggested Eyebrow Shapes for Each Face Shape in Chapter 9.

Note that some women will be able to wear more than one eyebrow shape. Others will be more restricted if they have a less common length or shape. Whatever the case may be, make sure that the length and thickness are proportionate to her features.

8. After making the shape selection, hold the template to the client's eyebrow and fill in the brow using pencil or eyebrow powder. Repeat the fill-in on the other side. Give the client a mirror to see the results. If the client is pleased with the shape of the eyebrow and requires hair removal outside the shape, proceed with hair removal as outlined in the Hair Removal Using the Template as a Guide section. If you are going to perform hair removal using the brow perfecting strip, proceed to the Hair Removal Using a Brow Perfecting Strip as a Guide section.

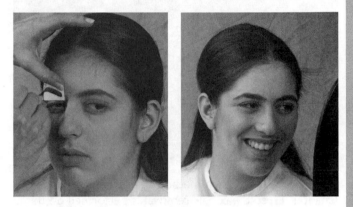

Filling in the client's brow helps create the newly designed shape and causes uneven brows to become symmetrical. The goal, if possible, is to have the client grow in the brow hairs where the fill-in is needed. Tell your clients not to remove any brow hairs at home but to continue to have that done in your salon. Explain that if their brow hairs do grow in and they do not inadvertently remove them, they will enjoy the benefit of a wonderfully designed brow shape that requires little or no fill in.

Step-by-Step: Hair Removal Using the Template/Brow Powder Fill-in as a Guide

1. Use an orangewood stick, an eyebrow brush, or a similar instrument to gently move unwanted hairs away from the newly filled-in brow shape. You can do this by separating or parting the hairs that do not have eyebrow powder on them from those that do have powder on them.

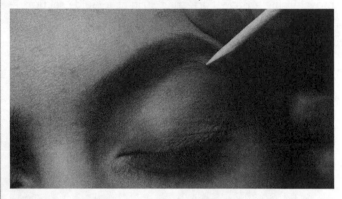

2. Perform the chosen method of hair removal (in Chapter 11, soft wax hair removal is performed on this client).

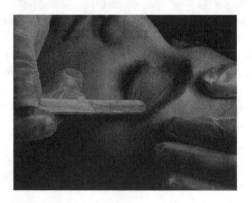

3. If the client requires a brow setting product, apply it gently to the brow hairs. Be careful not to touch the skin that has been affected by hair removal.

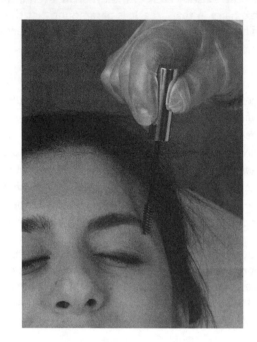

Step-by-Step: Hair Removal Using the Brow Perfecting Strip as a Guide

Once you have chosen the shape on the template, find the same exact brow shape on the brow perfecting strip. Some manufacturers use a coding system to help the user match the template to the strip that bears the same eyebrow shape.

1. Remove the eyebrow powder you applied in Step 8. Use a nonoily, fragrance-free eye makeup remover.

2. Take the inner, eyebrow-shaped part of the strip and adhere it directly to the eyebrow. Adhere the arch area first, then smooth down the beginning point and ending point areas.

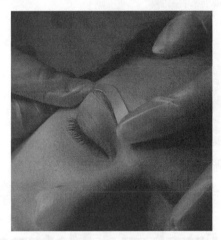

3. Use an orangewood stick, eyebrow brush, or similar object to separate the brow hairs that are to be removed from those that are under the strip.

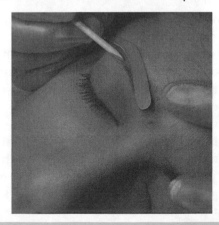

4. Perform the desired hair removal on hairs surrounding the strip. If you are waxing the eyebrow area, be careful not to get any wax underneath the brow perfecting strip.

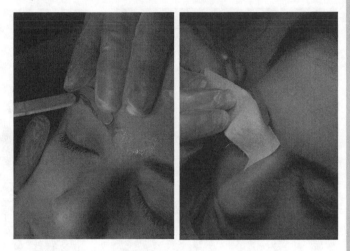

5. After the hair removal is complete, remove the strip from the eyebrow by pulling gently in the direction of the hair growth, from the inner corner, outward toward the ear. If you remove the strip correctly, you will not remove any brow hairs.

6. Using the outer part of the strip or the template, fill the brow in again using the desired brow colors to attain perfect symmetry.

7. If the client needs to use a brow setting product, apply it to the eyebrow only. Be careful to avoid areas that have been affected by hair removal.

8. The client will enjoy the remarkable transformation in her appearance from before her brow enhancement makeover (Figure 10–4) to after (Figure 10–5).

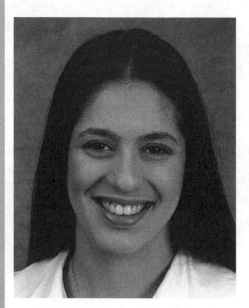

Figure 10–4   Before brow enhancement

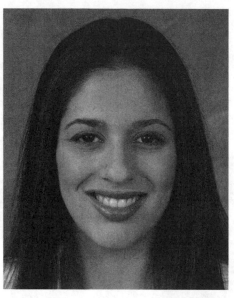

Figure 10–5   After brow enhancement

Professional Tip: In order to guarantee symmetry, the strips and templates must be held parallel to the floor when being used for fill-in. They are designed to fit the eyebrow only when they are held parallel. If you tip the template or strip in an attempt to match the existing eyebrow, you will not be able to match the degree of tipping on the other side, and, therefore, will not be able to attain symmetry. If you cannot match a particular template to a person's eyebrow without tipping it, then try another template.

The Freehand Method

Introduction

The freehand method is based on the application of the client's feature assessments and the rules of eyebrow placement and selection. Without the use of additional tools, the professional will use guidelines, coupled with her artistic abilities, to design an eyebrow shape for the client.

Room Setup, Tools and Supplies, and Client Preparation are the same for the Freehand Method as they are for the Template/Strip Method, except that you will not need the templates and strips to assist you.

Step-by-Step Procedure Using the Freehand Method for Total Eyebrow Creation

This client has relatively few existing eyebrow hairs (Figure 10–6). Therefore, the approach for this procedure is total eyebrow creation. Side notes are included for the brow enhancement approach so you can understand how it works with respect to the freehand method.

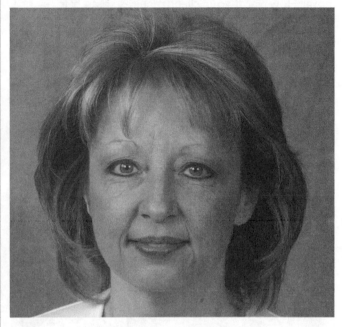

Figure 10–6   Before total eyebrow creation

1. Remove eyebrow makeup using eye makeup remover and a cotton pad.

2. Identify the client's eye set. Determine if the client's lip width is proportionate to her eyes.

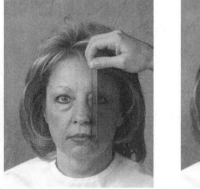
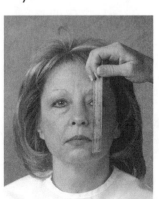

If you were performing brow enhancement using the freehand method, you would next perform the eyebrow assessment. This involves studying the length, texture, color, and excess hairs as outlined in the above procedure.

3. Study the color and tone of the client's hair and brow if any brow exists. Choose possible fill-in color options.

4. Using a ruler or measuring device, locate the ideal beginning and ending points for the brow. Lightly mark the desired beginning and ending points with an eyebrow pencil.

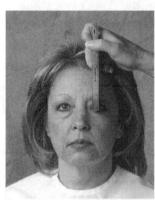
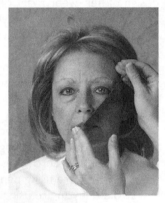

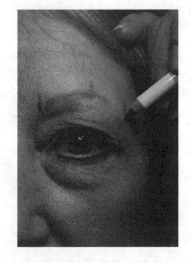

5. Decide on a flattering and well-fitting shape for the client. Table 10–1 lists the choices you will make and the features you will study to make them during the design process.

If you are performing brow enhancement, use the existing arch and the natural line of the eyebrow as the main guideline in creating the ideal shape. Then consider the elements listed in Table 10–1 to enhance the existing shape.

6. Ask the client how her eyebrows looked before she lost her hair. Refer to her eyebrow enhancement questionnaire to find out what she wants with respect to the design of her eyebrows. Confirm the client's face shape from your notes on her client profile and use Table 9–2 in Chapter 9 to help you design an attractive shape for her features. You may choose to sketch the eyebrow shape that you have determined is best suited for your client on the client profile so you can refer to it next time the client comes in.

7. Fill in the eyebrow based on the existing hairs (if there are any), the beginning and ending point measurements, and the eyebrow design you have created in Steps 5 and 6. If you are using pencil, fill in the shape using hair-like strokes. If you are using eyebrow powder, use upward and outward strokes. Make sure to complete the fill-in all the way to the correct ending point.

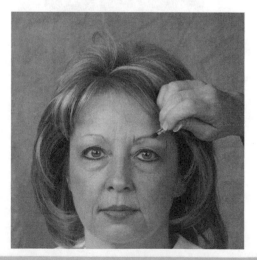

8. Give the client a hand mirror to show her the newly designed eyebrows.

9. In most total eyebrow creations cases, the client will not have much eyebrow hair and will not need hair removal. However, if your client requires some hair removal, perform that service at this point.

10. If the client needs to use a brow setting product for the sparse hair areas, apply it gently to the brow hairs. Be careful not to touch the skin that has been affected by hair removal.

11. The client will enjoy the remarkable improvement from before the total eyebrow creation (Figure 10–6) to after the work has been performed (Figure 10–7).

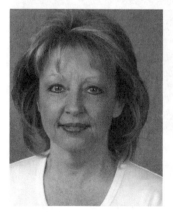

Figure 10–6 Before total eyebrow creation

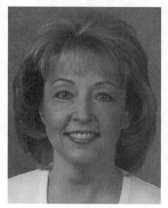

Figure 10–7 After total eyebrow creation using the freehand method

Practice Sheets

Use a pencil or pen, a ruler, and a "white out" product to enhance the eyebrows in Figure 10–8, 10–9, and 10–10. For Figure 10–10, you may wish to refer to Table 9–2, Suggested Brow Shapes for Each Face Shape in Chapter 9.

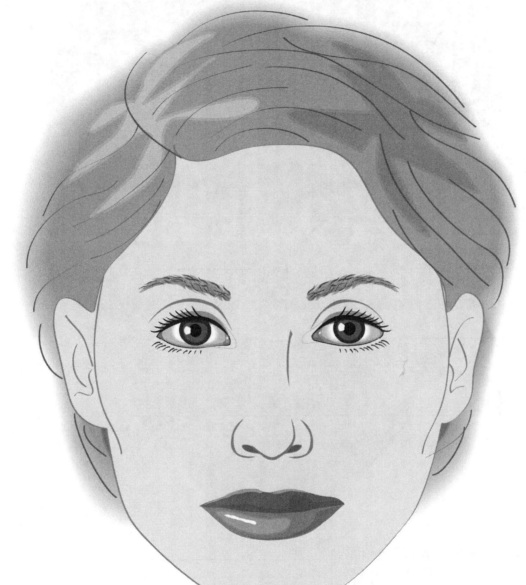

Figure 10–8

1. What face shape does this figure have? _____
2. Specify the eye set: close, well, wide _____
3. Use your ruler to locate the ideal beginning points. Which of the two is incorrect on this figure? _____ Pencil in that part of the eyebrow to make the correction.

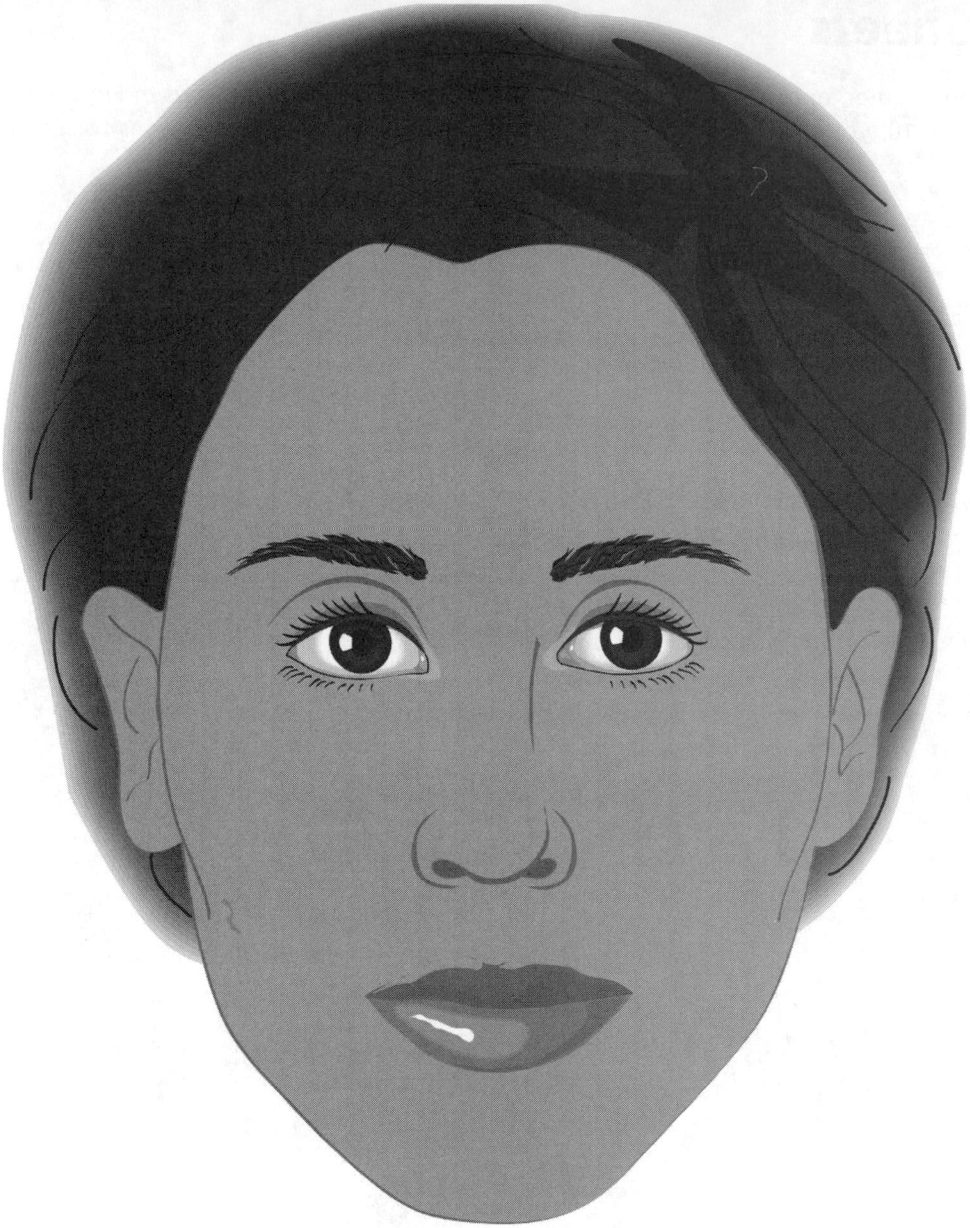

Figure 10–9

1. What face shape does this figure have? _____
2. Specify the eye set: close, well, wide _____
3. Locate the beginning and ending points using a measuring device. Are both points correctly placed?
   _____
4. Based on the eye set in this figure, is there a corrective technique that can be used? If yes, describe
   what you would do. _____
   _____
5. Use a pencil or a "white out" product to make the correction on the figure.

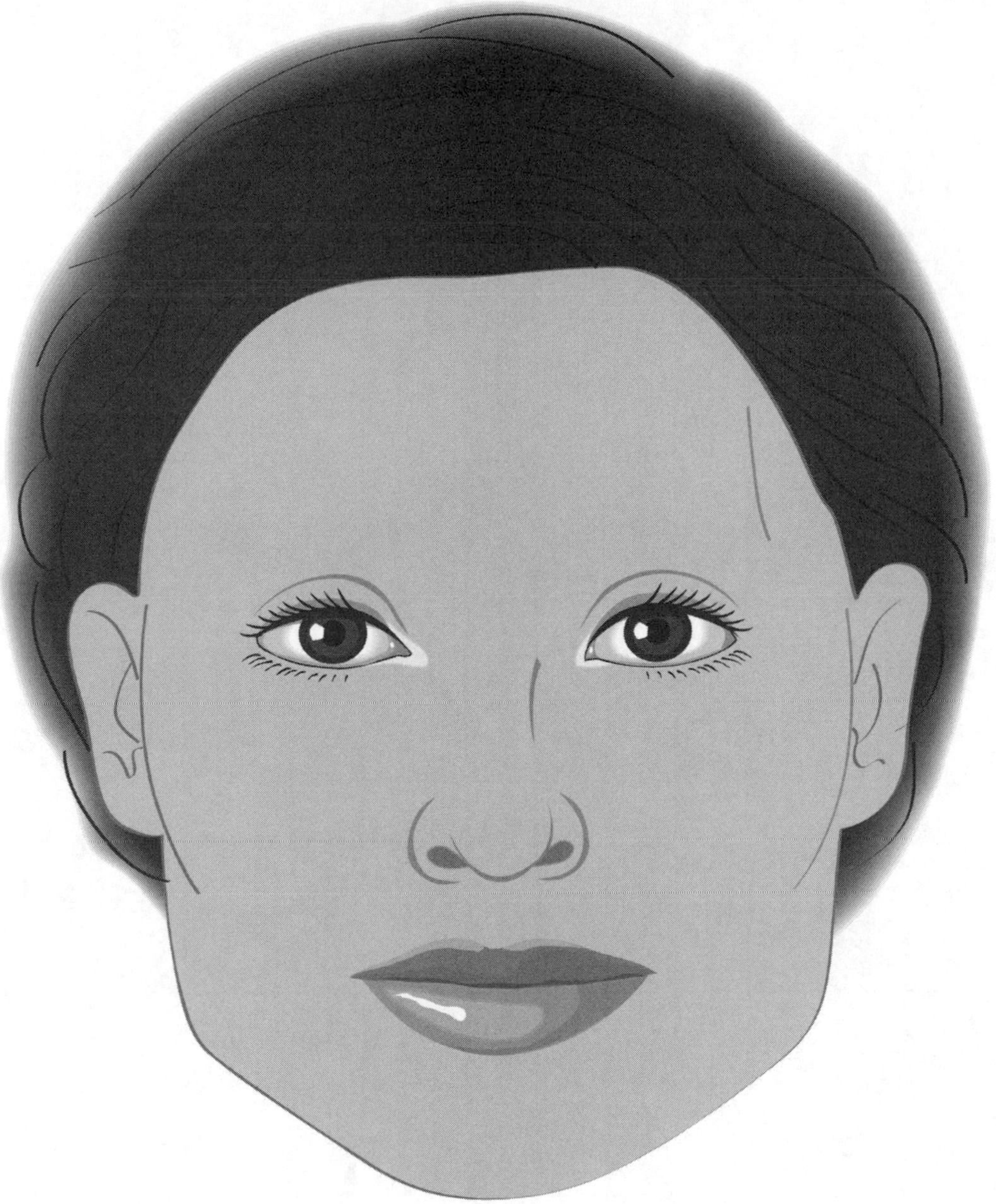

Figure 10–10

1. What face shape does this figure have? _____
2. Specify the eye set: close, well, wide _____
3. Based on you answer to Question #2, where should the beginning point of the eyebrow start? _____
   _____
4. Locate the beginning and ending points using a ruler or measuring device. Place a mark on the figure showing where they should be.
5. Draw an eyebrow shape that will look best on this face shape. Refer to Table 9–2 in Chapter 9 to help you decide on the optimal shape.

Chapter 11

HAIR REMOVAL FOR THE EYEBROWS

Learning Objectives

After reading this chapter, you should be able to:

1. Specify three reasons why hair removal performed on the brow area is more challenging than hair removal performed on other parts of the body.

2. Describe the basic structure of hair.

3. Explain the difference between epilation and depilation.

4. Discuss temporary versus permanent hair removal.

5. Understand and specify the contraindications of the various methods of hair removal.

6. List the different types of hair removal and the advantages and disadvantages of each method.

7. Discuss the difference between permanent hair removal and permanent hair reduction, and list the types of hair removal associated with each one.

Hair removal of the eyebrows is far more challenging than hair removal on other parts of the body. This is true because:

- the skin around the eye area is thinner than on other parts of the body
- the eyebrow area tends to be sensitive because large nerve trunks exist there
- the professional is expected to remove some, but not all, hair in the brow area, and leave an attractive shape that is created by the remaining hairs; even the slightest mistake involving the removal of a few extra hairs can make your client's brows uneven.

The purpose of this chapter is to familiarize you with the full range of hair removal options you can perform, or suggest others perform, for your client. To present the most up-to-date information, specialists in the different methods of hair removal share their expertise. To best learn from the information they present, it is helpful to first understand the difference between temporary versus permanent hair removal and the distinction between epilation and depilation. It is also helpful to recognize the different parts of the hair structure.

The Structure of Hair

Hair is composed of a hard protein called keratin. Keratin is produced from the hair follicle (Figure 11–1), which is a tube-like casing that houses the hair. The hair shaft is the part of the hair that is above the skin and the hair root is below the skin, inside the follicle. When we remove hair "by the root," we actually mean that it is removed all the way down to the hair bulb, which is the rounded portion of the hair at its base.

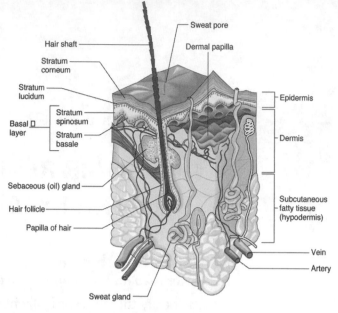

Figure 11-1   The structure of hair

Types of Hair Removal—Permanent versus Temporary and Epilation versus Depilation

Hair removal is classified in two ways. The first classification is temporary versus permanent hair removal. Electrolysis can lead to permanent hair removal if the treatments are done correctly and for the prescribed period of time. Laser hair removal can lead to a permanent reduction of hair if the treatment plan is followed. All other methods are considered temporary and must be done repeatedly.

The second classification is epilation versus depilation. Epilation is the removal of the hair below the surface of the skin, ideally by the root. Methods of epilation include tweezing, waxing, sugaring, threading, electrolysis, and laser hair removal. Depilation is removal of the hair at the surface of the skin. Methods of depilation include shaving and using depilatory creams. Unfortunately, when epilation is performed incorrectly, the result is that the client has been depilated, but has paid to be epilated. The goal is to remove the hair with the least amount of breakage possible so the client can enjoy a hair-free skin surface as long as possible.

The Methods of Hair Removal

Hair removal represents a relatively large percentage of revenue for the salon, in some cases as much as 50 percent. Waxing and tweezing have long been the predominant methods of hair removal performed in the salon. Many estheticians and cosmetologists are investigating and learning different techniques such as sugaring and threading to provide their clients with different alternatives. Beauty professionals can provide their clients with information and advice regarding hair removal services practiced by other professionals as they come to understand how these methods are performed. The methods of hair removal we will study are tweezing, waxing, sugaring, threading, laser, and electrolysis.

Tweezing

Tweezing Expert Rhonda G. Thomson (Figure 11–2) is the owner of Face and Body Essence Skin Care in

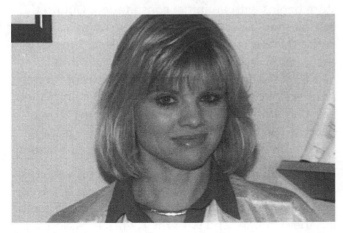

Figure 11–2   Rhonda G. Thomson, Esthetician and Educator

Fort Wayne, Indiana. Ms. Thomson has a degree in Business Administration and is a licensed esthetician, cosmetologist, and cosmetology instructor. She is a state educator for continuing education in cosmetology and an educational resources instructor for Ivy Tech State College. Ms. Thomson received her Advanced Certification in Esthetics from Purdue University. She has over 20 years experience in Business Administration and the Cosmetology Sciences.

With new clients, Ms. Thomson begins a typical tweezing session with a consultation. Once the consultation and design phases are completed, a tweezing session proceeds as follows.

1. Seat the client in a comfortable, slightly inclined position. The client may also be upright. The comfort of the client and the ease of completing the task should be the guideline.
2. Prepare the client by placing a towel across her shoulders or having her wear a disposable neck wrap and cape to protect clothing.
3. Tweezers, eyebrow brush, and trimming implements should be sanitized or sterilized and ready to use.
4. Cleanse your hands in the client's presence and put on disposable gloves, if you choose to wear them.
5. Cleanse the brow area with a disposable cotton pad soaked in cool water and sprayed with a mild antiseptic lotion or toner. Do not use oil-based products, which can cause the tweezers to slide.
6. If the client is very sensitive or is averse to pain, you can use professional Ice Globes to slightly numb the area.
7. Trim any long eyebrow hairs.
8. Working with an area about one inch of skin at a time, Ms. Thomson uses her thumb and index finger to gently hold the skin taut. Hair removal is performed by tweezing in the direction of the growth.
9. When tweezing is complete, place a cold, wet cotton pad on the area. Use a few drops of astringent on the pad to soothe the tweezed skin.

According to Ms. Thomson, there are few possible reactions one can expect from tweezing. "Ingrown hairs are not likely. In fact, tweezing is usually a remedy for ingrown hairs." Also, it is not necessary for clients to stop using any medications or topical creams before tweezing is performed on them.

Waxing

Waxing Expert Lori Nestore (Figure 11–3) is CEO of Eva's Esthetics in Oakland, California. Ms. Nestore is a licensed cosmetologist and has been a waxing specialist for 30 years. She is an internationally renowned speaker and consultant, and has become known as the "Wax Queen" for her speed and efficiency in performing hair removal with wax. In 1999, Ms. Nestore was awarded the Educator of the Year award at the Chicago Mid-West Beauty Show. She oversees the day-to-day operations of Eva's Esthetics while continuing her speaking and educational pursuits at trade shows, on television talk shows, and in various other venues.

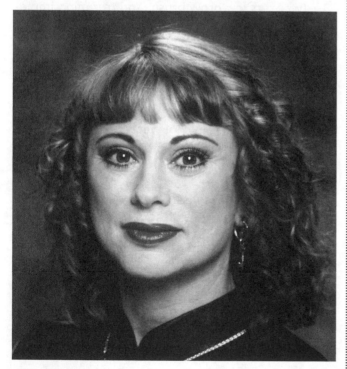

Figure 11–3 Lori Nestore, a.k.a., the Wax Queen and CEO of Eva's Esthetics

Waxing is the most common method of hair removal in the salon or spa environment. Differentiating between the types of waxes can be quite confusing because they are classified in many ways, such as:
- hard wax versus soft
- cold wax versus hot (or warm)
- strip wax versus stripless

Hard wax is most often stripless, but can be applied hot or cold (room temperature). Soft wax is always removed with a strip and is either warm or hot. There are cold waxes on a strip, even though "strip" waxes are generally associated with warm wax. It is easy to see why making the distinction between different types of waxes is not so simple. In addition, wax manufacturing companies often use the strip versus stripless differentiation because it is more absolute in terms of how it used.

Ms. Nestore prefers the traditional distinction of hard and soft for the different types of waxes. She defines and uses each as follows. Hard wax is heated to approximately 105°F and is applied thickly and removed without a strip. This type of wax is perfect for sensitive areas that also have coarse hair. These areas include the face, underarms, and bikini. Soft wax is also heated but is applied in a very thin layer, then removed with a strip. It is suitable for large body parts such as the legs, back, chest, and arms.

A typical eyebrow hair removal session with Ms. Nestore begins with an initial consultation. During the consultation, Ms. Nestore decides on an appropriate and attractive brow shape for the client. She has the client lie down for eyebrow hair removal, and for hair removal on all parts of the body except on the arms and shoulders. She trims the brow hairs if they are long. Nestore uses hard wax on the eyebrows because she believes it removes the coarse brow hairs more effectively with less trauma to the skin.

Her technique to effectively remove eyebrow hair is as follows. "Pick up a small amount of wax (the size of a large pearl) at the very end of the spatula. Holding the skin tight and with the client's eyes closed, apply the wax starting under the thickest part and spread it out to go past the end of the brow. The wax is spread in the direction of the hair growth. Use enough pressure to get the wax all the way down into the skin; don't just set it on top of the hair. Hard wax needs to have a thicker application than soft wax. You must create a slight ridge at the end where you will start the removal. Allow the wax to set for about 15 seconds. Hold the skin tightly at the end of the eyebrow. Flick (don't pick) the end to release the wax from the skin. Remove the wax in one quick motion, in the direction opposite the hair growth, keeping the hand close to the skin. Apply pressure for a second or two to calm the area." After the hair removal has taken place, she applies a blend of essential oils that she formulated strictly for the face.

Quickness and accuracy best describe how Lori Nestore performs and teaches the waxing service. "Slap that wax on and rip it off," are the words she uses to emphasize the main benefit of this type of hair removal: "quickness." She believes hair removal of the eyebrows should take about two minutes once the shape has been decided on in the consultation. Nestore never tweezes, but recommends that her clients let the shorter hairs grow in so they can be waxed during their next visit.

The following are additional tips provided by waxing expert Lori Nestore.

- make sure the client has a three-week hair growth before she is waxed
- have the client come back every three to four weeks for the next hair removal session
- your client will be clean (hair-free) much of the time once she gets past the initial three months of waxing

In addition to Ms. Nestore's teachings and advice, it is essential to consider the different contraindications to waxing (Table 11–1).

TABLE 11–1. WAXING CONTRAINDICATIONS

Drug/Condition	Precautions
Accutane	Do *not* wax or perform any exfoliation, whatsoever. Skin is highly sensitive and dry. If the skin is exfoliated—which includes waxing—it can be pulled off easily. Waxing can be resumed after a year of discontinuing the drug. Check with the client's physician.
Retin-A	Do *not* wax or perform any exfoliation on areas receiving Retin-A. Normally, brow arching is permitted simply because Retin-A should never be placed that close to the eyes. Thus, it is permissible to perform an arch. But be sure to verify that the client has not used Retin-A. Client must discontinue the drug in the brow area for five days prior to waxing and not resume until five days afterward.
Antibiotics	Skin sensitivities may occur, as well as susceptibility to infection if the skin is broken. The pH and moisture content of the skin is altered. Cleanliness is vital when working on a client who is taking antibiotics. Their skin is photosensitive, so clients must wear sunblock.

(continued)

Drug/Condition	Precautions
Birth control or hormone replacement	Skin may be more sensitive, more photosensitive, and more susceptible to pigmentation. Pull carefully to avoid irritation.
Blood thinners, i.e., Coumadin	No waxing without a physician's authorization. Clients taking blood thinners can bleed easily.
Autoimmune diseases—lupus, AIDS	Do not wax.
Cancer therapy—chemotherapy, radiation	Do not wax.
Diabetes, phlebitis	Do not wax unless client receives a physician's authorization.
Areas to avoid	No waxing on eyelids, or inside the nose or the ear cavity. Do not apply wax to the nipples on a man or a woman.
Open lesions (acne), cold sores, cysts, boils, growths, inflamed skin, sunburn, peeling or broken skin, cuts, moles, warts, active herpes virus	Do not wax.
Exfoliators—salicylic acid, AHAs, enzymes, scrubs, dipilatory creams	Depending on skin type and condition, client should discontinue use three days prior to waxing. Resume after three to four days, depending on skin condition. Must not have used dipilatory cream for at least one week or more.
Postcancer—excess hair growth	Many patients have extra hair growth around the sideburn area. Client must obtain a physician's permission to begin waxing. Perform waxing very carefully and gently. Follow with a cooling and soothing application.
Stimulants such as alcohol and caffeine	Skin tends to be more sensitive.
Smoking	Capillaries may be dilated and the skin may be more sensitive.
Severe sun exposure and tanning beds	Do not wax on any sunburned skin. Skin must be healed from sun lesions. Do not wax if the client has been in a tanning bed within the past 24 hours. The use of tanning beds is *never* recommended.

While Ms. Nestore uses hard wax to remove unwanted eyebrow hair, others prefer to use soft (warm or strip) wax. The following list of supplies, set up instructions, and step-by-step procedural example will provide you with guidelines and suggestions for performing soft (strip) wax hair removal to the eyebrows.

Using Soft (Strip) Wax to Remove Unwanted Eyebrow Hair

CHECKLIST OF SUPPLIES NEEDED TO PERFORM A SOFT (STRIP) WAX PROCEDURE TO REMOVE UNWANTED EYEBROW HAIR

Client Protection
___*towel, headband, or bobby pins to pull hair away from the face*
___*covering for client: either a towel for the chest area or a disposable neck wrap and client cape*
___*gloves (latex-free in case of allergy)*

Brow Trimming
___*eyebrow brush/comb*
___*sanitized or sterilized nippers or scissors*

Product and Supply Preparation
___*paper towels*
___*powder (corn starch, baby powder, or powder specifically formulated by wax manufacturer)*
___*shaker for the powder*
___*prewax lotion or antiseptic such as witch hazel*
___*wax removal lotion (can also use baby oil or petroleum jelly to remove wax residue or to remove wax that accidentally adheres to hair or skin)*
___*after-wax lotion (usually contains aloe or other soothing ingredients)*
___*cotton balls or pads*
___*eyebrow brush/comb or orangewood stick to part hair between the line of hair to be removed and the hair to remain*

Hair Removal Instruments
___*wax warmer/heater*
___*wax*
___*wax applicator (popsicle stick, orangewood stick, or spatula)*
___*precut muslin or pellon strips*
___*tweezers*
___*tissues or cotton balls to deposit tweezed hairs*

The Results
___*handheld mirror to show the client the results*

Set-Up Checklist for the Soft Wax Procedure

___**1.** Sanitize the esthetic chair, the sink, and all work areas using sanitizing solution in a spray bottle. Wipe with paper towels.

___**2.** Set up your work area. Lay out a paper towel. On the paper towel, place the following items: corn starch or powder; cotton balls; wax applicator sticks; prewax or antiseptic lotion; after-wax lotion, wax removal lotion, baby oil, or petroleum jelly; sanitized or sterilized tweezers; tissues, precut muslin, or pellon strips.

___**3.** Prepare the client's hair and draping accessories.

___**4.** Heat the wax to the desired temperature as specified by the manufacturer.

Figure 11–4 shows the areas of the eyebrows that can be waxed and provides a suggestion of the order in which to wax those areas (numbered one through five). You can wax the different areas in any order you choose, as long as all areas requiring hair removal are waxed.

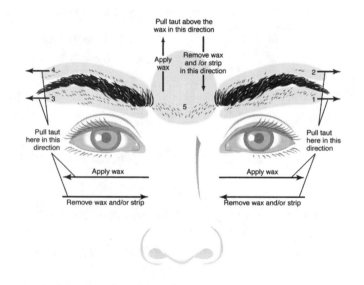

Figure 11–4   Eyebrow hair removal areas (direction to apply and remove wax is indicated by the arrows)

The Soft Wax Procedure

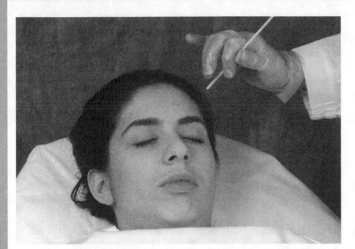

1. The eyebrow design has been completed for this model. Her new shape has been selected and she is ready for the hair removal phase.

2. Prepare the client for the wax procedure. The client can either be sitting or reclined with her hair pulled back from her face and her clothing protected with either a towel or a cape. Wash your hands in the presence of the client. If you choose to wear gloves, put the gloves on.

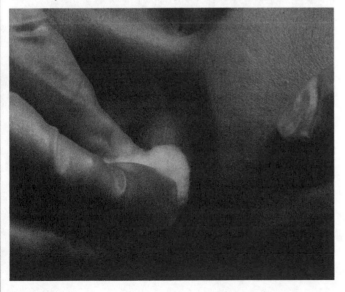

3. With a cotton ball, apply prewax lotion to the area to be waxed.

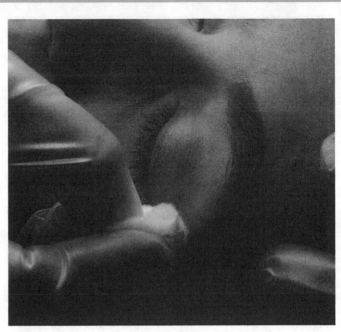

4. Dab a cotton ball into the powder and lightly apply the powder to the area(s) to be waxed. Avoid getting the powder into the eyes. The powder helps to dry the skin, allowing easier application of the wax. It also helps you more easily see the eyebrow hairs.

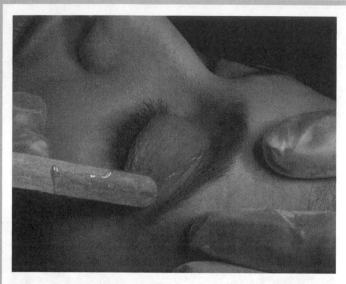

5. Dip the spatula or stick into the wax. Apply a thin coat of wax from the inside, under the thickest part of the brow, spreading outward in the direction of the hair growth. Discard the stick or spatula and never "double dip" a spatula into the wax.

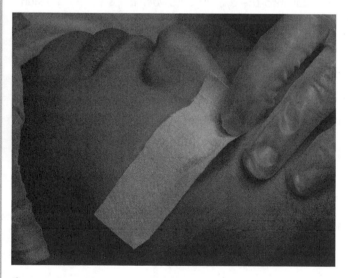

6. Lay the pellon or muslin strip on the wax. Smooth the strip in the direction of the hair growth until the wax partially seeps through and is visible.

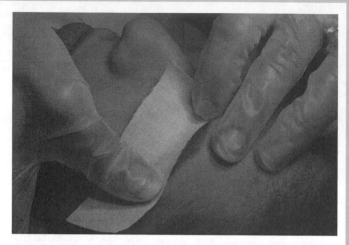

7. Hold the skin taut at the outer edge where the last portion of the wax was applied. Grab hold of the strip in preparation for removing it.

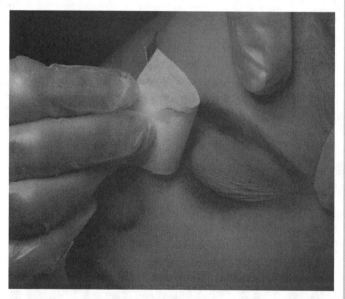

8. Remove the wax with a quick pull in the opposite direction of the hair growth. Do not pull the strip and the wax straight up. Instead, keep the hand close to the skin during the removal of the wax.

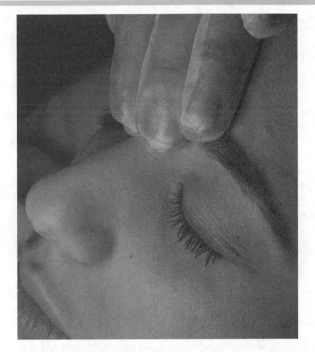

9. Immediately apply pressure with your finger(s) to the newly waxed area to lessen the pain.

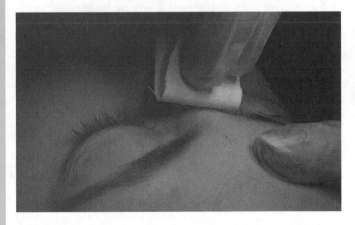

10. Proceed to wax all areas of the eyebrows until the unwanted hair is removed.

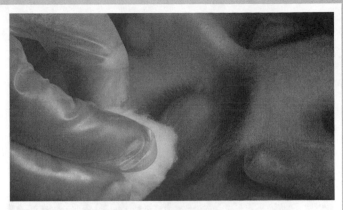

11. Using a cotton ball or a Q-tip, apply wax removal lotion, baby oil, or petroleum jelly to remove any residual wax.

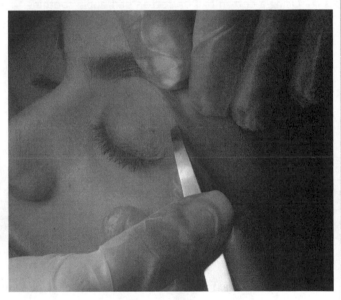

12. If you wish to remove any remaining hairs, you can tweeze them with sanitized or sterilized tweezers. Tweeze the hairs in the direction of the growth while pulling the skin taut in an outward direction. Deposit the removed hairs on a cotton pad or a cotton ball, or use a tissue that is wound neatly around your finger.

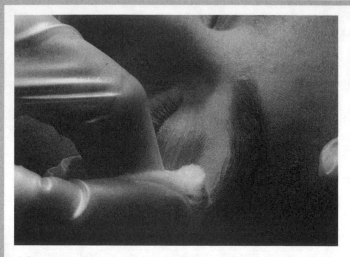

13. Using a cotton ball or cotton pad, apply soothing after-wax lotion to the waxed areas.

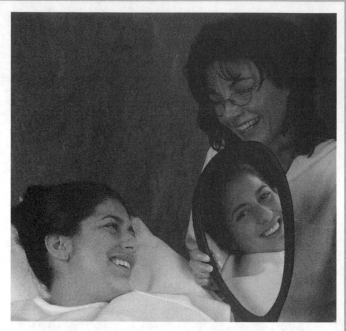

14. Allow the client to sit up if she was reclined during hair removal, and give her a hand mirror so she can see the results.

15. Remove the client's head towel or headband. The client's eyebrows are well-designed, attractive, and free of unwanted hair.

Wax Bands

As an alternative to conventional waxing methods, some hair removal specialists prefer to use cold wax on a strip. An example of one such product that is sold to salon professionals is a cold wax band impregnated with milk (Figure 11–5).

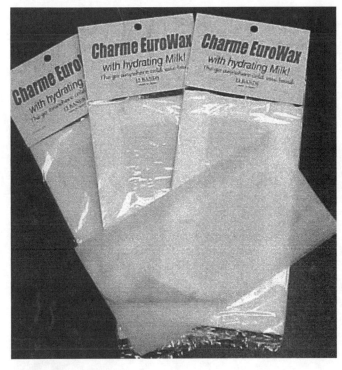

Figure 11–5   Cold wax bands

According to Antonio Olivera, Vice President of Charme International, "Impregnated wax bands are disposable, which is optimal for sanitary considerations. They cannot burn the client's skin because the wax is cold and is warmed by rubbing the bands between the hands. Additional equipment is not needed to heat the wax, which makes the wax bands portable. They contain milk, which is hydrating and calming to the skin. The bands are made of a very high-quality material which helps prevent irritation."

The procedure for using the cold wax bands is similar to the procedure for using soft (strip) wax. The wax band is cut to the desired shape (Figure 11–6), rubbed to soften the wax, and then applied in the direction of the hair growth. Like conventional waxing methods, the cold wax band is removed against the direction of the hair growth.

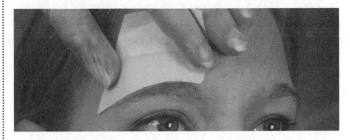

Figure 11–6   The cold wax band is cut to the desired shape before using

Sugaring

Sugaring Expert Lina Kennedy (Figure 11–7) is President of Alexandria Professional Body Sugaring™.

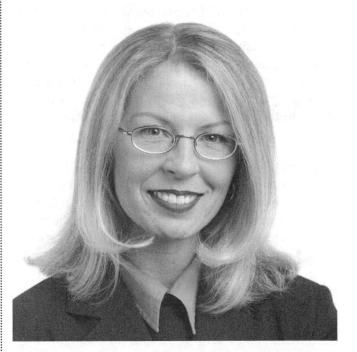

Figure 11–7   Lina Kennedy, President, Alexandria Professional Body Sugaring

Lina Kennedy has been an Alexandria Professional Body Sugaring (APBS) practitioner since 1991. In 1995, Ms. Kennedy obtained exclusive international distribution rights for the products and then purchased the manufacturing rights in 1996. With this, she owned the entire professional line of Alexandria Body Sugaring™. She has recently been featured on FOX television and in numerous publications worldwide including *101 Celebrity Style*, *Les Nouvelle Esthetique*, *DaySpa Magazine*, *SalonSense*, and *Beauty Times Magazine*.

Sugaring is a traditional hair removal method practiced throughout many generations. It is difficult to pinpoint when sugaring was first performed, but it is believed to have originated in the Middle East many centuries ago.

Each sugaring product contains different components, depending on the company that manufactures them. Alexandria's sugaring products are 100 percent natural, edible, and water-soluble. They do not breed bacteria because the paste has such a high concentration of sugar. Some companies offer a wax-based product and add sugar to it. This is not a sugar hair removal product in its purest form and this type of product will have the same results as a waxing product. However, if your intent is to use a product that is different from wax, make sure the ingredients contain only sugar and other natural, nonwax, nonresin ingredients.

A typical eyebrow hair removal session with an Alexandria Professional Body Sugaring™ practitioner begins with the client consultation. If it is the first consultation, the client fills out a client record card and learns about the contraindications of and possible reactions to sugaring.

After a suitable eyebrow shape is designed, the client is asked to lie down. The sugar paste is preheated and is kept at a temperature that is slightly cooler than lukewarm so there is no chance of burning the client's skin. The process of removing the hair is as follows.

1. Apply an antimicrobial skin cleanser to the area using a cotton pad.
2. Apply a toner-like antiseptic to the area. Ms. Kennedy uses "Essential Tonic" (Figure 11–8), that possesses antimicrobial, antiseptic, antifungal, antiviral, and anti-inflammatory properties.

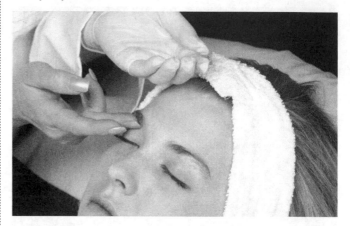

Figure 11–8   Apply an antiseptic toner

3. Apply "Vertal 6 Drying Powder" to the area. Gently pat it onto the skin area to be treated (Figure 11–9).

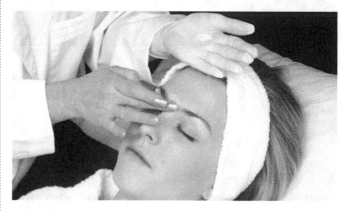

Figure 11–9   Apply a drying powder to prepare area for the sugar paste application

4. Take a small amount of paste with the index finger and apply to the area requiring hair removal, from the outer (Figure 11–10) to the inner eye (Figure 11–11). The sugar paste is always applied in the opposite direction of the

hair growth and is always removed in the direction of the hair growth. This is opposite to the way wax is applied and removed.

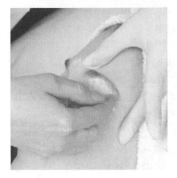
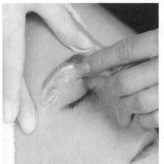

Figure 11–10   Sugar paste is applied AGAINST the direction of hair growth, beginning at the outer part of the brow

Figure 11–11   Finishing the application of sugar paste

The practice of applying the sugar paste against the growth of the hair is called, "moulding." Moulding is the process where the sugaring paste wraps itself around the hair shaft and makes the hair more pliable. Simultaneously, the sugaring paste seeps below the mouth of the follicle and lubricates the hair root inside the follicle. This process provides maximum ease of extraction with minimal discomfort.

5. Remove the sugaring paste by flicking it in the direction of the hair growth (Figure 11–12). This is done while holding the skin taut with the index finger and thumb of the support hand. After both brows are done, both beneath and above the brow, remove unwanted hair in between the brows using the same procedure (Figure 11–13).

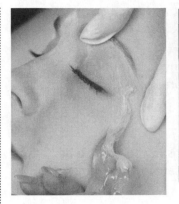
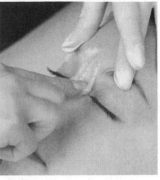

Figure 11–12   Removing (flicking) the sugar paste. Sugar paste is removed in the direction of the hair growth

Figure 11–13   Hair removal with sugar paste, in between the brows

6. Immediately following the removal of the hair, swipe the area again with an antiseptic toner.

7. The final step is to treat the area with a soothing lotion. Ms. Kennedy recommends Alexandria's "Restore Hydrating Lotion" (Figure 11–14), which contains chamomile extract and other soothing ingredients. The client will be free of excess eyebrow hair with minimal skin irritation (Fig. 11–15).

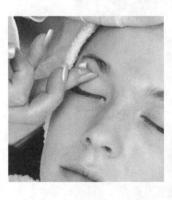

Figure 11–14   Calming and soothing the sugared areas with a hydrating lotion

Figure 11–15   The client after a sugaring hair removal session

As with waxing, there are situations in which a client should not undergo a sugaring procedure. Do not sugar clients if they:

- are using Retin-A or any Retinol treatment
- have recently undergone a heavy peel (one- to five-day peel)
- are using Vitamin C topical products in the area
- are using Accutane
- have specific conditions in the area to be treated such as new scars, sunburned skin, warts, or skin lesions

Threading

Threading Expert Shobha Tummala (Figure 11–16) is the owner of the Just Shobha™ salon in New York and creator of the Shobha™ Threading Introduction Program (TIP). Ms. Tummala has a degree in Electrical Engineering from Michigan State University and has an MBA from Harvard Business School. She is the owner of Just Shobha™, a salon in the heart of SoHo in New York City.

Threading is an ancient hair removal technique. Its earliest practices are difficult to trace, but it is thought to have originated many centuries ago in Arabia. Threading is a practice that is traditionally taught by family members or friends to one another, and is passed on from generation to generation. As a young girl growing up in India, Ms. Tummala learned how to thread from one of her cousins. Back then, she did not realize the value of the craft. She later rediscovered the practice on one of her trips back to India. While there, she visited a local salon and got perfectly shaped arches after having been told by countless waxing professionals that she could not. She has been a threading enthusiast ever since, leading to her creating TIP through which she has taught thousands of professionals the art and science of threading.

Shobha™ certified threaders use different types of thread based on the type of hair to be removed (Figure 11–17). They use a polyester/cotton thread on the eyebrows and upper lip, a silk/cotton thread

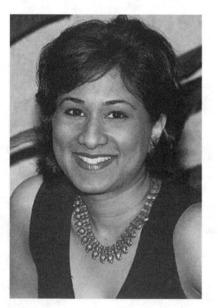

Figure 11–16   Shobha Tummala for Eyes of the World, Inc.

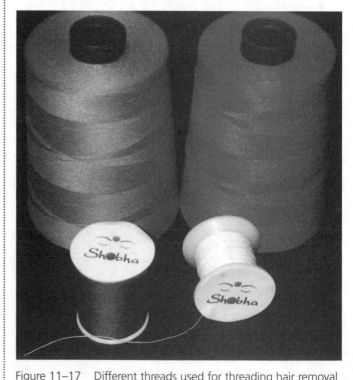

Figure 11–17   Different threads used for threading hair removal

for other facial hairs, and a 100 percent cotton thread on other parts of the body. Ms. Tummala currently imports her threads from India and makes them available to salon professionals.

The benefits of threading are numerous. According to Ms. Tummala, "Threading is the best hair removal option that exists for removing facial hair. It cannot be matched in its sensitivity, precision, cleanliness, or swiftness of results. Threading utilizes specially chosen thread, which is twisted and pulled along the area of unwanted hair, lifting it directly from the follicle. Threading works very well for parts of the body that are very sensitive or require precision like the brows, upper lip, sideburns, and other facial areas."

A typical eyebrow hair removal session with a certified threader begins with a client consultation. During this time, the practitioner and the client discuss the desired outcome in terms of eyebrow shape. If it is the client's first threading session, they are given a brief description of the procedure and what they can expect from the results. It is unlikely that the client will have a breakout or skin irritation, but that possibility is also explained. Finally, the client is asked to refrain from using any alphahydroxy, glycolic, or any other type of acid product for 24 hours after the threading is completed.

After the initial consultation is completed, the client lies down on the esthetic chair for the procedure. After sanitizing her hands, the threader prepares the eyebrow area by wiping it with alcohol to remove any oil, dirt, or makeup that may be on the skin. Some threaders then apply talcum powder to a cotton ball and gently dab it on the area to be treated. Spreading the powder in the area decreases the chance of the skin getting caught in the thread.

The threader begins removing the hair by deftly twisting the thread using one of three different methods. In the first method, the threader holds the end of a thread in her mouth while using both hands to pull it taut (Figure 11–18). The thread is quickly wound around an individual hair, similar to how a rope is lassoed around a post. The thread is then skillfully twisted and pulled to extricate the hair from its follicle. The process is repeated until all unwanted hair is removed. Because of the swiftness of the craft, a typical eyebrow hair removal session takes only about 10 minutes.

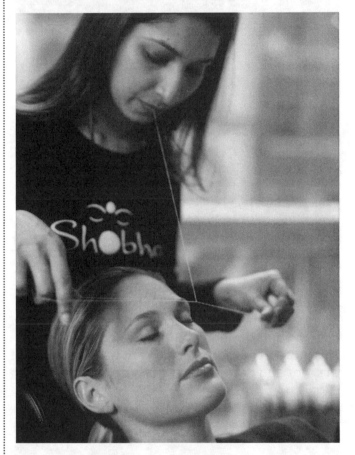

Figure 11–18   The thread is skillfully twisted and the end is held in the threader's mouth

A second variation of threading includes using the threader's neck to manipulate the loose ends of the thread instead of the mouth. The third method involves using just the hands to wind the thread (Figure 11–19). The latter two methods do not use the mouth. Some state Cosmetology Boards prohibit using the mouth for sanitary reasons while other states have no regulation against it.

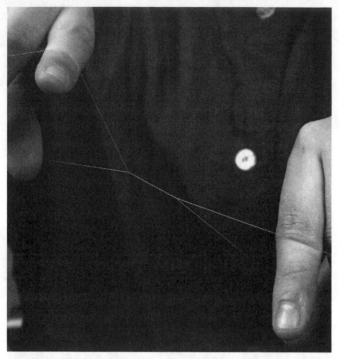

Figure 11–19   The thread is skillfully twisted, using only the hands for this method.

For the method using only the hands, the threader captures the hair in the point of the "V" while opening and closing the other side of the thread. This movement causes the hairs to be removed by the root and become captured onto the thread (Figure 11–20).

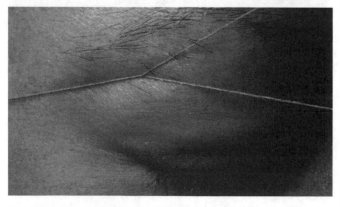

Figure 11–20   Threading the eyebrow hairs using the hands–only method

After all unwanted hair is removed, the professional applies rose water toner to a cotton ball or pad and gently wipes the treated area. Rose water is known to reduce redness and swelling. The threading session is finished, and again, generally takes about 10 minutes once the consultation is complete. The client is encouraged to return every three to five weeks to keep the brow area well shaped and free from hair.

Laser Hair Removal

Laser Hair Removal Expert Omeed M. Memar, M.D., Ph.D. (Fig. 11–21) is Medical Director of the Academic Dermatology & Skin Cancer Institute in Chicago, Illinois. Dr. Memar graduated from the prestigious M.D., Ph.D. program at the University of Texas Medical Branch. His Ph.D. is in the field of immunopathology of the skin. He completed his residency at the University of Illinois at Chicago where he was trained by leaders in the field of dermatology, dermatopathology, hair biology, and dermatologic surgery. Dr. Memar is certified by the American Board of Dermatology and the American Society for Mohs Surgery.

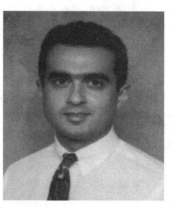

Figure 11–21   Omeed Memar, M.D., Ph.D., dermatologist and dermatologic surgeon

Laser hair removal is a relatively new technique that Dr. Memar believes has revolutionized hair removal. Dr. Memar prefers laser to other hair removal methods because the sessions are shorter and the number of sessions required by the patient to attain permanent hair reduction is fewer. In addition, Dr. Memar has found that the likelihood of folliculitis formation is much less. Folliculitis is an inflammation of the follicle that is caused either by an irritation or by bacteria that has entered the follicle.

Laser hair removal is based on selective thermolysis. In this process, the laser light is attracted to darker colors because they absorb greater wavelengths of light. When the laser is cast toward the skin, the dark colored hairs attract the laser, which generates heat as a result of the wavelength absorption. This heat leads to microscopic damage of the melanin in the hair bulb (root). In order to avoid damaging the skin's melanin, which is pigment that gives the skin its color, the newer lasers have a cooled tip. The tip prevents the melanin from becoming heated and causes further preferential heating of the deeper melanin, which is in the hair bulb.

The first laser-assisted hair-removal device was marketed in 1996. Since then, many different devices have been manufactured and sold. Among them is the Nd-Yag 1064nm Lyra (Figure 11–22), made by Laserscope, which is used by Dr. Memar.

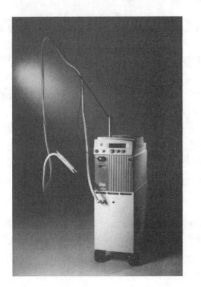

Figure 11–22   Laserscope's LYRA Nd–Yag laser hair removal system

Before the procedure begins, the treatment room is prepared. The equipment is sanitized and the supplies are prepared. A typical eyebrow hair removal session with Dr. Memar begins with a client consultation. The initial consultation is thorough as Dr. Memar:

- goes over the consent form that includes a description of the procedure, a description of other alternative procedures for hair removal, and a description of the advantages of laser hair removal. The patient signs the necessary consent forms.
- informs the patient that the most dangerous part of laser eyebrow hair removal is possible damage to the eyes if the laser light comes in contact with the eye. The laser operator must wear protective eye gear, and clients must wear protective eye shields in addition to keeping their eyes closed during the entire process.
- informs the patient that the eyebrow area requires an average of seven sessions of laser hair removal at six-week intervals.
- discusses the pain sensation with the client and describes it as the stinging feeling that occurs when someone snaps a rubber band on the skin. He explains that the amount of sensitivity varies per client, based on nerves and pain threshold levels.
- shares with clients how lasers work. He informs them of the rare instances when scarring can occur.
- provides the client with a list of do's and don'ts for before and after laser hair removal.

Also during the consultation, the client may request the application of a topical cream that will lessen the discomfort. If so, he has the client apply Ela-Max-5 cream to the area, under a plastic wrap, one hour prior to the procedure.

Once an eyebrow shape has been selected, the hairs to be lasered are shaved, leaving the remaining hairs to form the newly designed eyebrow. The patient is situated in an upright position. The eyebrow area is cleansed with alcohol, taking care to remove all cosmetics. The eyes are covered with protective eye shields and the client is cautioned to keep her eyes closed during the procedure. Dr. Memar then performs the laser hair removal on the shaved areas. The process takes about 15 minutes for both brows. After the hair has been lasered, he applies a hydrocortisone ointment to soothe the area. He recommends that the patient apply sun block with an SPF of 30 or higher at all times.

Laser hair removal requires specialized training from an experienced practitioner or from the manufacturer of the equipment that is used. Some states now require laser education and licensure before practicing laser hair removal. Each state's regulations vary, making it necessary to investigate your state's regulations.

It is important to understand that the procedure is not always effective for people with light-colored or white brow hairs because the laser light will not be absorbed into the lighter color hair. The lack of attraction means those hairs will not receive the heat in order to destroy the bulb. Some laser systems use a carbon-based cream to attract light to fair hair. Results vary as to the effectiveness of this approach. Suffice it to say that this new method of hair removal is gaining popularity quickly. As time goes on, new developments will improve the methods and results for greater client satisfaction.

Electrolysis

Electrolysis is the process of permanently removing hair by using electricity to destroy the hair follicle. According to *Milady's Standard Comprehensive Training for Estheticians*, there are three methods of electrology.

1. Galvanic, which uses direct current and causes chemical decomposition of the hair follicle.
2. Thermolysis, which utilizes high-frequency current to produce heat and destroys the hair follicle.
3. Blend, which combines both systems, sending current through a fine needle or probe.

If a client requests information from you regarding your opinion and experience regarding electrolysis,

you will want them to know that it is currently the only form of permanent hair removal available. Improvements in laser technology and other inventions may spawn other permanent methods in the future, but for now, electrology stands alone in its ability to provide permanent hair removal. Your client should also know that the process of permanently removing unwanted hair usually requires weekly or bi-weekly electrology sessions over a time period of six months to one year, with possible subsequent touchups.

At this time, there is no national standardization for certification to practice electrolysis. Training requirements, testing standards, and certification requirements vary from state to state. A little more than half of all states require electrologists to be licensed. Some states require practitioners to be licensed under the state's Medical Board as a Cosmetic Therapist (CT), which involves many hours of training and testing. Other states require little or no training or testing. The International Guild of Professional Electrologists maintains a list of licensed and certified electrologists, and can assist you and your clients in finding a reputable professional to perform this service.

Comparing the Different Methods of Hair Removal

Deciding which method of hair removal the professional and the client prefer is based on many important factors. Table 11–2 presents a thorough analysis of the different aspects of hair removal such as an appropriate price to charge the client and the minimum length the hair should be in order to effectively perform each type of hair removal. Table 11–3 provides a concise listing of advantages and disadvantages of each type of hair removal.

As a beauty professional, it is incumbent upon you to understand the different hair removal options available to the client, whether or not you are able to perform each one. You will be better equipped to educate your clients so you can help them make the choices that best serve them.

TABLE 11-2. COMPARISON OF THE DIFFERENT METHODS OF HAIR REMOVAL FOR THE EYEBROWS

Hair Removal Method: Epilation vs Depilation, Permanent vs. Temporary	Minimum Hair Length Required for Effective Hair Removal	Average Length of Time to Perform Hair Removal from the Eyebrow Area after Consultation is Performed	Recommended Price Range for Simple Eyebrow Hair Removal Service (Note: The recommended one-time fee for "Eyebrow Design" is $20–$50 and higher)	Who Can Legally Perform this Service? Is Certification Required?
Tweezing Epilation, Temporary	1/16 of an inch or less	10–30 minutes	$13–$15/session	Licensed beauty professionals
Waxing Epilation, Temporary	4/16 (one-quarter) of an inch or longer; that is, approximately 3–4 weeks of hair growth	2–10 minutes	$10–$20/session	Licensed cosmetologist or esthetician. Some states like New York have waxing licensure
Sugaring Epilation, Temporary	1/16 of an inch or 2–4 days after shaving	10–20 minutes	$12–$17/session	Licensed beauty professionals. Training and certification by the manufacturer is recommended
Threading Epilation, Temporary	1/16 of an inch. If you can pick the hair up with tweezers, then it can be removed by a threading practitioner	Approximately 10 minutes	$20–$30/session	Licensed beauty professionals. Training is necessary in order to learn the skills and techniques
Laser Epilation, Permanent Hair Reduction	None. Since the laser works on the hair bulb, the hair shaft (the hair above the skin) is not necessary. The area is shaved and the shaved area is then lasered.	Approximately 15 minutes	$300–$600/session. (Note: price varies per office). Seven sessions every six weeks is often recommended.	Doctor or licensed beauty professional under the supervision of a doctor. Some states now require a minimum number of education hours. Varies per state.
Electrolysis Epilation, Permanent Hair Removal	1/16 to 2/16 of an inch	Often 30 minutes; some electrologists use 20-minute or 45-minute blocks of time	$25–$75/session	Varies by state. Currently, 31 states require some type of certification. Regulated by the Medical Board in some states.

Hair Removal Method: Epilation vs. Depilation, Permanent vs. Temporary	Advantages	Disadvantages
Tweezing Epilation, Temporary	Inexpensive; requires only tweezers; allows for accuracy because you only remove the hairs you want to remove; no need to wait for regrowth of hair.	Not permanent; slow; some consider tweezing painful and because it is so slow, it is painful for a long time.
Waxing Epilation, Temporary	Very quick; easily accessible to the beauty professional; excellent for areas that have a lot of hair to be removed.	Not permanent; unwanted skin removal can occur if professional uses wrong product or procedure; hot wax can possibly burn the client's skin; must have 3–4 weeks of hair growth for effective removal; may irritate skin.
Sugaring Epilation, Temporary	Only 1/16 of an inch (2–4 days) of hair growth is needed for effective hair removal; true sugar paste is kept and applied lukewarm so there is no chance of burning the skin; sugaring paste doesn't adhere to live skin cells and thus will not accidentally remove skin; less irritating than a resin wax; sugar paste is easily removable with water.	Not permanent; must be done by a trained practitioner to achieve the desired results; if done incorrectly, can cause breakage of hairs.
Threading Epilation, Temporary	Only 1/16 of an inch (2–4 days) of hair growth is needed for effective hair removal; no artificial waxes or chemicals are applied; therefore, threading is not as irritating to the skin as other methods may be; relatively quick; a high degree of control and precision allows practitioner to remove hair to create intended eyebrow design; disposable piece of thread is sanitary.	Not permanent; must be done by a trained practitioner to achieve the desired results; if done incorrectly, can cause breakage of hairs.
Laser Epilation, Permanent Hair Reduction	Can lead to permanent hair reduction; relatively quick; excellent for large areas of the body that have unwanted hair; hair growth is not necessary because the area is first shaved, then the shaved area is lasered.	Some consider lasers to be painful (feels like a rubber band snapping on skin) but depends on pain threshold; expensive compared to other methods of hair removal; must be done by a reputable, qualified, and trained professional to be effective.
Electrolysis Epilation, Permanent Hair Removal	If recommended treatments are undertaken, can lead to permanent hair removal (this is the only method that can attest to that advantage); hair can be as short as 1/16 of an inch to effectively perform the service.	Some consider electrolysis to be painful, but again, this depends on pain threshold; can be costly over time; length of treatment generally six months to one year for permanence; must find a qualified, capable electrologist to perform the service correctly; if incorrectly done, can cause the skin to become discolored.

REFERENCES

D'Angelo, J., Lees, M., Dean, P. S., Miller, E., Dietz, S., Zani, A., & Hinds, C. 2003. *Milady's standard comprehensive training for estheticians.* Clifton Park, NY: Delmar Learning.

Kennedy, L. (2000). *Alexandria professional body sugaring reference guide* (3rd ed). Welland, Ontario, Canada.

Chapter 12

OTHER EYEBROW ENHANCEMENT SERVICES

Learning Objectives

After reading this chapter, you should be able to:

1. Define permanent makeup.

2. List alternate names for "permanent makeup."

3. Specify the characteristics of a client who might benefit from permanent makeup application.

4. Define tinting.

5. Describe the brow characteristics of a client who could benefit from having her eyebrows tinted by a professional.

In addition to hair removal, other services can be performed to enhance the eyebrow. Some of the more unique services that can be performed on the brows are dermaplaning, brow plugging, and false eyebrow application. In this chapter, we have included a discussion of two other services performed on the eyebrows: tinting and permanent makeup.

Permanent Makeup

Permanent makeup, also known as micropigmentation or tattooing, is the process of applying colored dye into the dermis. The permanency of this service means that the permanent makeup artist should be exceptionally proficient in eyebrow design. If not, a client could suffer years of anguish if an ill-designed brow is etched onto their forehead. When the eyebrows are well designed and permanent makeup is correctly applied, the client who receives this service will benefit greatly.

Any person who pencils or powders in their eyebrows every day is a perfect candidate for permanent makeup. The client will gain personal freedom from having to repeat this laborious task every day. The client will no longer have to worry about having uneven eyebrows or the possibility of her eyebrows rubbing off at the wrong time. Combining proper eyebrow design techniques with skilled permanent makeup application can ultimately increase the client's self-esteem and confidence.

Permanent Makeup

Permanent Makeup Expert Rose Marie Beauchemin (Figure 12–1) is the owner of The Beau Institute of Permanent & Corrective Cosmetics, and a Permanent Cosmetics Specialist and Instructor. Ms. Beauchemin has been in the beauty industry for over 30 years. As a licensed cosmetologist and salon owner, she marketed her own line of private label cosmetics, as well as hairpieces and wigs. She has taught wardrobe engineering workshops throughout the country to improve the appearance of executives

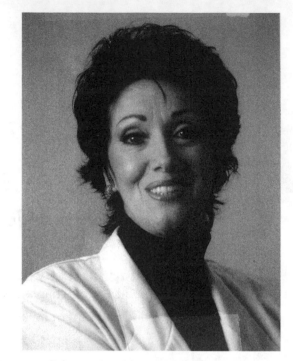

Figure 12–1   Rose Marie Beauchemin, Director of Education of The Beau Institute of Permanent Cosmetics and The Brow Hospital, LLC

and their wives for corporate giants such as McDonald Corporation, Subaru of America, and the Four Seasons Hotel. Ms. Beauchemin has owned her permanent makeup practice for over 10 years and became a permanent makeup artist after hearing her clients consistently say, "If I could only take you (Beauchemin) home with me!" after she performed a regular cosmetic application. She was exhilarated by the idea that she could make this possible for her clients through the art of permanent makeup.

Permanent makeup is thought to have evolved from the art of body tattooing, which has been traced back to the Ice Ages. According to Ms. Beauchemin, "Today we see the more familiar and obvious connection to its Asian roots. In ancient China, only royalty were adorned with tattooed eyebrows, to clearly separate them from the masses. You will see this exemplified in the paintings on glass of the ancient dynasty emperors and empresses of China. Eventually, the appeal of this defined brow trickled down to the common folk and remains very popular in the Asian countries. In the early 1980s, a brilliant ophthalmologist and visionary, Dr. Gioro Angres, realized that today's busy woman would appreciate the benefits of this ancient art. Dr. Angres brought this technique to Hollywood, where he began to teach professionals how to perform this work."

When it was initially practiced, permanent makeup was performed on only a few, select individuals. It has since evolved into a widely practiced form of cosmetic application throughout the United States and the world.

Permanent Makeup Equipment, Supplies, and Sanitation

There are many different manufacturers of products and equipment, each with its separate set of techniques used to perform the service. The list of supplies and equipment necessary to perform the work of micropigmentation is vast. Each practitioner uses his preferred system, which differs in many aspects from the type(s) of needles (disposable or nondisposable), all the way to the different types and colors of pigments available. According to Ms. Beauchemin, "There are various needle groups and sizes for the different procedures such as eyeliner, lips, and eyebrows. Needles are also configured differently for various techniques such as hair simulation or shading. The needles are truly the paint brushes of the face for a permanent cosmetic practitioner."

In order to use the equipment and supplies in a safe manner, it is of the utmost importance to follow all sanitation and safety procedures. "Because the needles penetrate the client's skin, it is common to have trace amounts of blood present. The practitioner absolutely must wear procedural gloves, gowns, and safety glasses. The client needs

to be covered with a poly-backed bib. The needles must be sterile and as many of the supplies that can be disposable should be disposable. Finally, room cleanup must be done with a separate set of gloves that are for cleanup purposes only."

The Preprocedure Consultation for Permanent Makeup

Before the procedure begins, a client consultation is performed. During this consultation, which can take place a week or more before the actual procedure, the process is explained in detail, along with the possible side effects and product use warnings.

Ms. Beauchemin is vehement that, "Practitioners should never tell their client to stop using a medication, not even aspirin. This could prove to be a reckless and negligent thing to do, since this is a medical decision and requires medical clearance from the client's physician." However, a client is asked to refrain from using topical creams that contain Retin-A, glycolic, or alphahydroxy acids at least 15 days prior to the procedure and during the healing period.

Preprocedure photographs are taken of the client wearing her makeup. Next, the makeup is removed to evaluate the tone and subtone of her skin. This analysis assists the practitioner in choosing attractive pigment colors. Eyebrow measurements are taken and the eyebrow shape is designed. Excess eyebrow hair is removed either by waxing or tweezing, if necessary.

The Permanent Makeup Procedure

On the day of the procedure, the client comes in, is greeted, and begins to fill out the necessary paperwork. A topical numbing cream is applied to the area while the client completes the paperwork. The numbing cream is applied, as needed, throughout the procedure to alleviate discomfort. The eyebrow design that was created during the preprocedure consultation is recreated on the client's brows by filling them in. Once the client gives the final approval of the eyebrow design, the practitioner mixes the pigment and the procedure begins.

Ms. Beauchemin describes the procedure as follows. "The pen is dipped into the mixed pigment, where it is held in a reservoir. The pigment is released as the pen makes contact with the skin. As the machine touches the skin, it begins to drop pigment that is pushed or injected into the dermal tissue by the needle or needles. The pen is held at a 45° angle and the pigment goes into the top layers of the dermal tissue at a depth of 1.25 millimeters to 1.75 millimeters. The practitioner must be careful not to allow the pigment to go too deep into the subcutaneous layer, where some color would quickly be carried away by the lymphatic system. This would create an eyebrow with a murky appearance."

After the work is finished, a light redness and swelling usually occurs in the immediate area, but will last only one or two days. Vaseline is applied after the procedure to protect the skin. There is an eventual fading of the tattooed area, which occurs more quickly in the eyebrow area, because the sebaceous activity and exfoliation of the face are more rapid there than on other parts of the body. Also, the face is constantly exposed to the elements, which hastens the fading process.

The length of time is takes to apply permanent makeup to the eyebrow area after the consultation is completed ranges from one-half hour to upward of two hours. The cost varies, based on location and work performed, and should be in the range of $300 to $600 per session. Permanent makeup to the brow can last anywhere from three to five years if it is performed correctly.

Figure 12–2 shows a photograph of a woman before permanent makeup was applied to her eyebrows and Figure 12–3 shows the same woman after the procedure was performed. The remarkable difference in her appearance provides evidence of the advantages of correctly applied permanent makeup.

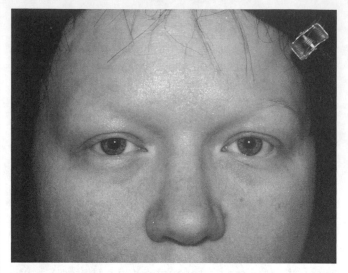

Figure 12–2   Before—Client before permanent makeup is applied to the eyebrows

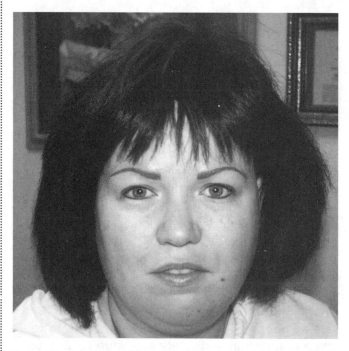

Figure 12–3   After—Client after permanent makeup is applied to the eyebrows

Before and After of Permanent Makeup courtesy of The Beau Institute.

Eyebrow Tinting

A client may wish to change her brow hair color to a darker or a lighter color. There are different methods of temporarily changing the color of a person's eyebrows, some of which are permissible in the salon while others are not. Unfortunately, many clients would like to change their brow color, but there are very few safe and legal options available to the salon professional for that purpose. Some professionals either do not understand the regulations regarding these services or they simply disregard them.

The methods that are too dangerous to perform in the salon are bleaching of the eyebrows to lighten them and applying haircolor to match the head hair color. State Cosmetology Boards have regulated against providing these services in the salon or spa environment.

The only method of temporarily changing the color of the eyebrows that can be offered and performed in the salon in all states is to use eyebrow powders. Eyebrow powder must be made of certain, high-quality ingredients in order to change the color and adhere to the brow and skin. Not all eyebrow powders stay on as long as they should. The disadvantage to this way of changing the brow color is that the powders must be applied every day. The only other permissible option available is tinting.

Eyebrow Tinting

Tinting Expert Karen Wallace (Figure 12–4) is an Educator and Instructor of Esthetics and Cosmetology at Grace College of Cosmetology in Middleburg Heights, Ohio. Ms. Wallace is a licensed cosmetologist and instructor. She owned her own salon for over 20 years. She is currently the head instructor for cosmetology and an instructor of esthetics for Grace College of Cosmetology.

Tinting is the process of using safe, nonaniline derivative ingredients that deposit color to the brow

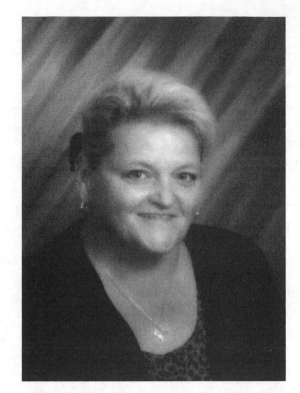

Figure 12–4 Karen Wallace, Head Cosmetology Instructor and Esthetics Instructor

hairs when mixed and applied according to the manufacturers' directions. "Tinting can last as long as four to eight weeks or longer," Ms. Wallace states. "Tinting is a wonderful option for the client whose brow hair color is too light, but, yet, has enough brow hairs to be able to design a beautiful brow shape."

Ms. Wallace warns, "Tinting of the eyebrows is a service that is permissible in the salon in some states, but not in others. It is necessary to check your state's Cosmetology Board to learn about the regulations pertaining to tinting before you perform the service." You must follow all of the manufacturers' instructions when using any tinting product.

LIST OF SUPPLIES NEEDED FOR AN EYEBROW TINTING PROCEDURE

Client Protection

___towel, headband, or bobby pins to pull hair back and away from the face

___covering for the client's clothing such as a disposable neck wrap and a client cape

___gloves (latex-free in case of allergy)

Tinting Products/Other Supplies

___cotton

___cotton balls or pads

___petroleum jelly

___clean dish with warm, soapy water

___clean dish with warm, clear water

___handmade cotton-tipped applicators (made by taking a small wooden stick and winding a small piece of cotton tightly around one end)

___extra wooden toothpick-like sticks

___tinting solution #1

___tinting solution #2

___tint stain remover

___two clear glass dishes or cups

SET UP FOR THE TINTING PROCEDURE

1. Sanitize the treatment area.

2. Set out all products and supplies. So you do not confuse the two clear tinting solutions when they are dispensed, pour solution #1 into a clear dish or cup and set the bottle next to it. Do the same for solution #2.

3. Make the handmade tint applicators. The manufacturer often provides the toothpick-like sticks to wind the cotton around. Q-tips can also be used as the tint applicator.

The Tinting Procedure

1. The eyebrow design and hair removal processes should be done before the tinting procedure. Ms. Wallace recommends waiting at least 24 hours after hair removal has been performed before performing the tinting service. If there are no signs of irritation after that time, then you can proceed.

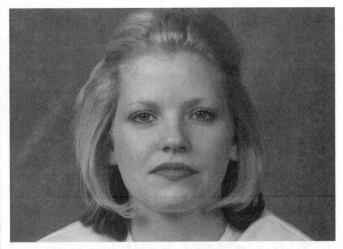

2. The client should be sitting upright to lessen the chance of solution seeping into her eyes. Clean both brows with a cotton ball dipped in soapy water. Ms. Wallace adds, "Do not use a skin cleanser to wash the brows and brow area because the oils in the cleanser may prevent the tint from adhering to the brow hair." Rinse the area with a cotton ball that has been soaked in clear water.

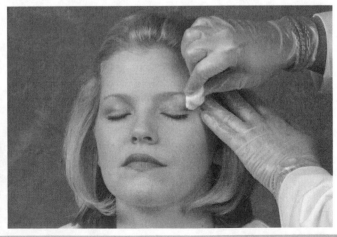

3. Use a disposable spatula to remove petroleum jelly from its container. Apply a thin coating to the areas surrounding the eyebrow hairs to protect the skin. Do not allow the jelly to touch the brow hairs or the tint will not adhere to the brow hair.

4. Use a handmade applicator and apply the first solution (solution #1) to the top side of the eyebrow beginning at the inner corner of the brow and ending at the outer corner. Ms. Wallace recommends the next step to provide even tinting coverage. "Do not neglect to tint the underside of the brow hairs. Use a wooden stick to lift the brow hair while using the handmade applicator to apply solution #1 to the underside, beginning from the outer corner of the brow and ending at the inner corner of the brow." Do not let the solution touch the skin. This procedure allows application of the solution to both sides of the hair. Apply solution #1 to the top and underside of the other eyebrow. You will not see a color change during the application of the first solution. Allow the solution to dry for three minutes.

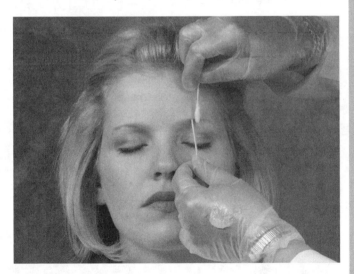

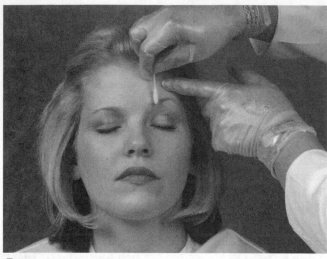

8. In order to eliminate the stain remover residue, wash the area again with soap and water using cotton balls. Gently dry the area.

9. The client will enjoy her newly tinted eyebrows that will provide additional emphasis and focus on her beautiful eyes.

5. Apply the second solution (solution #2) the same way you applied the first solution. As soon as the second solution is applied, you will see the color change. Be careful to apply the minimal amount needed so the solution does not run into the eyes. Allow the solutions to dry together for one minute.

6. Wash the brows and surrounding area with a cotton ball soaked in soapy water. Rinse the area using a cotton ball soaked in clear water.

7. Use a cotton-tipped applicator to apply the tint stain remover to any places where the skin was accidentally stained.

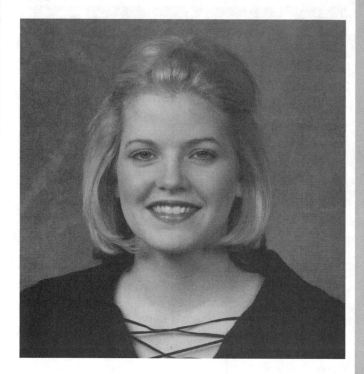

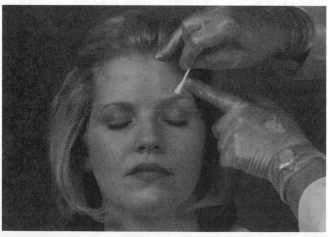

The tinting process can take as little as 10 minutes to perform and can provide the client with a temporary reprieve from having to fill in light eyebrow hairs every day. The average charge for a tinting service can range from $15 to $20 and higher.

Chapter 13

CASE STUDIES: EYEBROW DESIGN IN PRACTICE

Learning Objectives

After reading this chapter, you should be able to:

1. Assess a client's facial and eyebrow features, and fill out her client profile.

2. Use the information on the eyebrow enhancement questionnaire and the client profile to perform careful and thoughtful "eyebrow design."

3. Discuss how and why you arrived at a specific "eyebrow design" for a client's given features and existing eyebrow condition.

The following case studies present a sampling of clients with different eyebrow problems. As you work through each case study, you will learn how to perform "eyebrow design" in a systematic way, increasing your knowledge and confidence with each new client.

In the first three case studies, all of the forms you learned about are used and you will have the chance to fill out the client profile on your own. You will compare your client profile to ours and learn from any differences. You will see the re- markable transformation that occurs as a result of careful and thoughtful "eyebrow design."

The fourth case study is your chance to design the eyebrows for a client on your own. You will fill out all of the forms and "pencil in" or "remove" the brow hairs on the client (on the page) in the book, using pencil and a "white out" product.

After you complete the case studies, you will be ready to take the Master Eyebrow Specialist test.* With consistent practice and your Master Eyebrow Specialist certification, you will be able to confi- dently design the "perfect eyebrow" for all of your clients.

Instructions for
Case Study #1, #2, and #3

Examine the face and eyebrows of each client shown in the case studies, along with her responses on her eyebrow enhancement questionnaire. Fill out a blank client profile for each case study client and compare it to the one we completed for each client. Reconcile and learn from any differences. (Note: When you complete a client profile, there are certain questions you will be unable to answer such as "Type of Work.") Study the other forms, learn from the recorded information, and understand how the assessments translate into the newly designed eyebrows.

To become a certified Master Eyebrow Specialist, go to www.perfectbrow.com to take the test online. You can also download and print the test. For any questions regarding your certification, contact Adriel, Inc. at 1-800-273-7126.

CASE STUDY #1:
Sparse Eyebrows

Eyebrow Enhancement Questionnaire

Client Name: _Anita Jamrah_   Date: _2/15/03_

A. Your Eyebrows

   1. What do you like about your eyebrows?
     shape

   2. What would you like to change about your eyebrows?
     The arch

B. Your Health and Medications

   3. Have you used Accutane in the last seven years? _No_

   4. Are you currently using Accutane? _No_

   5. Are you currently using Retin-A? _No_   Renova? _No_

   6. Are you currently taking blood thinners such as Coumadin? _No_

   7. Do you use any of the following: Salicyclic acid, alphahydroxy acids, enzymes, scrubs, depilatory creams, vitamin C creams? If so, please list and describe your frequency of use.

   8. Do you have: ❑ Diabetes   ❑ Cancer   ❑ High Blood Pressure   ❑ Acne   ❑ Phlebitis   ❑ Autoimmune Diseases such as Lupus   ❑ Sunburn

   9. Have you ever had an adverse reaction after hair removal? If yes, specify the type of hair removal and the adverse reaction you had.
     _No_

   10. Have you been in the sun or in a tanning bed within the last 48 hours? _No_

C. Your Preferred Method of Hair Removal

   11. What type of hair removal do you wish to have done today? _Wax_

I have answered all of the questions to the best of my knowledge. I understand that the professional may refuse to provide epilation services because of certain health conditions and that it is in my best interest if the service is not provided. I also understand that there may be swelling or irritation in the areas that are waxed or otherwise epilated. This is only a temporary condition.

Client's Signature _Anita Jamrah_   Date _2-14-03_

CLIENT PROFILE FOR EYEBROW ENHANCEMENT SERVICES

Name: _____ Date: _____

1. Face Shape: ☐ Round ☐ Long ☐ Square ☐ Oval ☐ Inverted Triangle or Heart ☐ Pear
   ☐ Diamond ☐ Hexagon

2. Circle zone(s) that is/are wide.   Upper   Middle   Lower

3. Circle zone(s) that is/are long.   Upper   Middle   Lower

4. Indicate client's eye set.   Close   Well   Wide

5. Overall size of features: Small   Medium   Large

6. Size of nose _____

7. Is lip width proportionate to eye width? ☐ yes ☐ no

8. Eye orientation: Almond   Even   Drooping

9. Color tone: Warm   Cool

10. Personality type: ☐ Natural ☐ Conservative ☐ Artistic ☐ Extravagant
    ☐ Relaxed/carefree ☐ Intense ☐ Demure ☐ Other

11. Age group: ☐ Twenties ☐ Thirties ☐ Forties ☐ Fifties ☐ Sixties or older

12. Type of work _____

13. Current condition of eyebrows

    _____

    _____

14. What features would the client like to cosmetically enhance?

    _____

    _____

15. Ideal length of eyebrow: ☐ 1^7/$_8$" ☐ 2" ☑ 2^1/$_8$" ☐ 2^3/$_8$" ☐ other

16. Other important information

    _____

    _____

CLIENT PROFILE FOR EYEBROW ENHANCEMENT SERVICES

Name: Anita Jamrah   Date: 2/15/03

1. Face Shape: ☐ Round ☑ Long ☐ Square ☐ Oval ☑ Inverted Triangle or Heart ☐ Pear ☐ Diamond ☐ Hexagon

2. Circle zone(s) that is/are wide.   (Upper)   Middle   Lower

3. Circle zone(s) that is/are long.   (Upper)   Middle   Lower

4. Indicate client's eye set.   (Close)   Well   Wide (slightly close set)

5. Overall size of features: Small   (Medium to Large)

6. Size of nose   Medium and well proportioned

7. Is lip width proportionate to eye width? ☐ yes ☑ no

Lips appear slightly wide in relation to the inside of the iris. Upon visual inspection, it is clear that the lips are not too wide for the face, but it is the client's close-set eyes that skew the results of the lip width test. To cosmetically correct this client's slightly close-set eyes, you can either start the beginning point barely outside the standard beginning point and/or make the arch further out than the halfway point along the brow.

8. Eye orientation: Almond   (Even)   Drooping

9. Color tone: Warm   (Cool)

10. Personality type: ☐ Natural ☐ Conservative ☑ Artistic ☑ Extravagant ☐ Relaxed/carefree ☐ Intense ☐ Demure ☐ Other

11. Age group: ☑ Twenties ☐ Thirties ☐ Forties ☐ Fifties ☐ Sixties or older

12. Type of work   Student

13. Current condition of eyebrows
Existing brows are too thin -- medium to thick shap would be more consistent with feature size. Existing brows are asymmetrical

14. What features would the client like to cosmetically enhance?
Make forehead appear less prominent either by changing hairstyle or by making the arch more prominent toward the center of the brow

15. Ideal length of eyebrow: ☐ 1⁷/₈" ☐ 2" ☑ 2¹/₈" ☐ 2³/₈" ☐ other

16. Other important information
The client does not want eyebrows that are "too thick." A medium thickness is suitable.

Name: Anita Jamrah   Date: 2/15/03

EYEBROW PRESCRIPTION FORM

In order to maintain beautiful, symmetrical eyebrows, the following items are recommended:

☐ Eyebrow brush/comb

☑ Tweezers

☐ Brow setting product

☑ Eyebrow powder in Dark brown, medium brown, auburn _____ colors

☐ Eyebrow pencil in _____ colors

☑ Eyebrow powder applicator stiff _____

☑ Template in 2 1/8"; arch slightly beyond mid-point; thin or medium thickness ___ shape

☐ Brow perfecting strips in _____ shape

☑ It is recommended that the client have waxing or tweezing _____ (type of hair removal) performed every ____4____ weeks.

You can schedule your next appointment before leaving today. We will call you to confirm.

(Your Salon Name)

(Salon Telephone Number)

Before

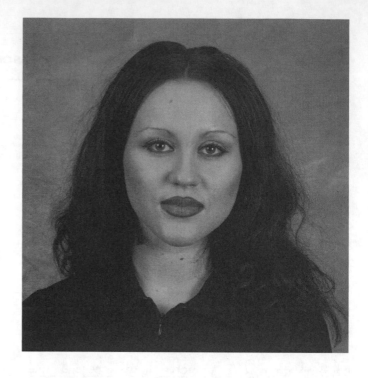

After

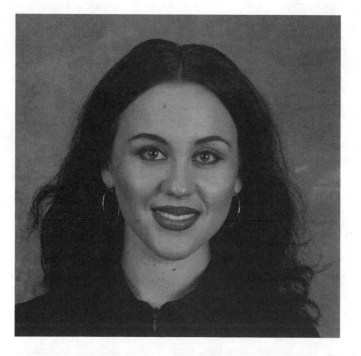

CASE STUDY #2:

Full Eyebrows

EYEBROW ENHANCEMENT QUESTIONNAIRE

Client Name: __Tina Deddonna__   Date: __2-21-03__

A. Your Eyebrows

   1. What do you like about your eyebrows?
      __I like the arch of my eyebrows__

   2. What would you like to change about your eyebrows?
      __I would like to change the length (impossible i know) but i do wish they were longer__

B. Your Health and Medications

   3. Have you used Accutane in the last seven years? __No__

   4. Are you currently using Accutane? __No__

   5. Are you currently using Retin-A? __No__   Renova? __No__

   6. Are you currently taking blood thinners such as Coumadin? __No__

   7. Do you use any of the following: Salicyclic acid, alphahydroxy acids, enzymes, scrubs, depilatory creams, vitamin C creams? If so, please list and describe your frequency of use.

   8. Do you have: ❑ Diabetes   ❑ Cancer   ❑ High Blood Pressure   ❑ Acne
      ❑ Phlebitis   ❑ Autoimmune Diseases such as Lupus   ❑ Sunburn

   9. Have you ever had an adverse reaction after hair removal? If yes, specify the type of hair removal and the adverse reaction you had.
      __Nair for facial hair removal. it burned me bad, i have sensitive skin also so that probably was the problem__

   10. Have you been in the sun or in a tanning bed within the last 48 hours? __No__

C. Your Preferred Method of Hair Removal

   11. What type of hair removal do you wish to have done today? __Wax__

I have answered all of the questions to the best of my knowledge. I understand that the professional may refuse to provide epilation services because of certain health conditions and that it is in my best interest if the service is not provided. I also understand that there may be swelling or irritation in the areas that are waxed or otherwise epilated. This is only a temporary condition.

Client's Signature __Tina Deddonna__   Date __2-21-03__

CLIENT PROFILE FOR EYEBROW ENHANCEMENT SERVICES

Name: _____ Date: _____

1. Face Shape: ❑ Round ❑ Long ❑ Square ❑ Oval ❑ Inverted Triangle or Heart ❑ Pear
   ❑ Diamond ❑ Hexagon

2. Circle zone(s) that is/are wide.   Upper   Middle   Lower

3. Circle zone(s) that is/are long.   Upper   Middle   Lower

4. Indicate client's eye set.   Close   Well   Wide

5. Overall size of features: Small   Medium   Large

6. Size of nose _____

7. Is lip width proportionate to eye width? ❑ yes   ❑ no

   _____

8. Eye orientation: Almond   Even   Drooping

9. Color tone: Warm   Cool

10. Personality type: ❑ Natural ❑ Conservative ❑ Artistic ❑ Extravagant
    ❑ Relaxed/carefree ❑ Intense ❑ Demure ❑ Other

11. Age group: ❑ Twenties ❑ Thirties ❑ Forties ❑ Fifties ❑ Sixties or older

12. Type of work _____

13. Current condition of eyebrows

   _____

   _____

14. What features would the client like to cosmetically enhance?

   _____

   _____

15. Ideal length of eyebrow: ❑ 1⅞" ❑ 2" ☑ 2⅛" ❑ 2⅜" ❑ other

16. Other important information

   _____

   _____

   _____

   _____

CLIENT PROFILE FOR EYEBROW ENHANCEMENT SERVICES

Name: Tina Deddonna   Date: 2-22-03

1. Face Shape: ❑ Round ☑ Long ❑ Square ❑ Oval ❑ Inverted Triangle or Heart ❑ Pear
   ❑ Diamond ❑ Hexagon

2. Circle zone(s) that is/are wide.   Upper   Middle   Lower
3. Circle zone(s) that is/are long.   (Upper)   Middle   (Lower)
4. Indicate client's eye set.   Close   (Well)   Wide
5. Overall size of features: Small   (Medium)   Large
6. Size of nose Small-medium
7. Is lip width proportionate to eye width? ☑ yes ❑ no

8. Eye orientation: (Almond)   Even   Drooping
9. Color tone: Warm   (Cool)
10. Personality type: ❑ Natural ❑ Conservative ☑ Artistic ☑ Extravagant
    ❑ Relaxed/carefree ☑ Intense ❑ Demure ❑ Other
11. Age group: ☑ Twenties ❑ Thirties ❑ Forties ❑ Fifties ❑ Sixties or older
12. Type of work Cosmetologist
13. Current condition of eyebrows
    Client has a full brow that requires some hair removal. The client has an artistic
    flair and prefers the highly arched brow.
14. What features would the client like to cosmetically enhance?
    The client wishes to maintain the appearance of her features while making her
    appearance a little more clean and groomed.
15. Ideal length of eyebrow: ❑ 1⁷⁄₈" ❑ 2" ☑ 2¹⁄₈" ❑ 2³⁄₈" ❑ other
16. Other important information
    This client wears bangs or some hair on her forehead most often. Therefore, it is
    esthetically correct if she chooses an arched, instead of a flatter brow shape.
    Because the client's existing eyebrow shape is well-suited, freehand eyebrow design can
    be easily performed to soften the arch and slightly thin out and clean up the
    eyebrow.

Name: _Tina Deddonna_____ Date: _2-22-03_____

EYEBROW PRESCRIPTION FORM

In order to maintain beautiful, symmetrical eyebrows, the following items are recommended:

☑ Eyebrow brush/comb

☐ Tweezers

☑ Brow setting product

☐ Eyebrow powder in _____ colors

☐ Eyebrow pencil in _____ colors

☐ Eyebrow powder applicator _____

☐ Template in _____ shape

☐ Brow perfecting strips in _____ shape

☐ It is recommended that the client have _Waxing_____ (type of hair removal) performed every _2-3_____ weeks.

You can schedule your next appointment before leaving today. We will call you to confirm.

(Your Salon Name)

(Salon Telephone Number)

Before

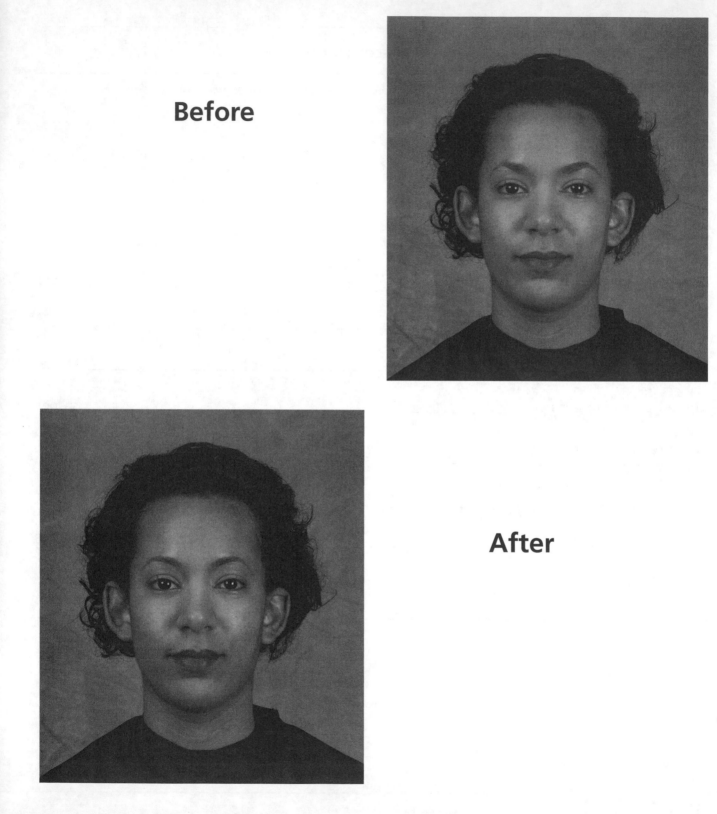

After

CASE STUDY #3:

Poorly Shaped Eyebrows

EYEBROW ENHANCEMENT QUESTIONNAIRE

Client Name: _Rosanna Stanfa_   Date: _2-22-03_

A. Your Eyebrows

    1. What do you like about your eyebrows?
      I like the darkness in color and the length.

    2. What would you like to change about your eyebrows?
      I would definitely like them to be thicker and more of an arch would be nice.

B. Your Health and Medications

    3. Have you used Accutane in the last seven years? _no_

    4. Are you currently using Accutane? _no_

    5. Are you currently using Retin-A? _no_   Renova? _no_

    6. Are you currently taking blood thinners such as Coumadin? _no_

    7. Do you use any of the following: Salicyclic acid, alphahydroxy acids, enzymes, scrubs, depilatory creams, vitamin C creams? If so, please list and describe your frequency of use.
      Clearasol astringent

    8. Do you have: ☐ Diabetes   ☐ Cancer   ☐ High Blood Pressure   ☐ Acne
      ☐ Phlebitis   ☐ Autoimmune Diseases such as Lupus   ☐ Sunburn

    9. Have you ever had an adverse reaction after hair removal? If yes, specify the type of hair removal and the adverse reaction you had.
      _no_

    10. Have you been in the sun or in a tanning bed within the last 48 hours? _no_

C. Your Preferred Method of Hair Removal

    11. What type of hair removal do you wish to have done today? _tweezing_

I have answered all of the questions to the best of my knowledge. I understand that the professional may refuse to provide epilation services because of certain health conditions and that it is in my best interest if the service is not provided. I also understand that there may be swelling or irritation in the areas that are waxed or otherwise epilated. This is only a temporary condition.

Client's Signature _Rosanna Stanfa_   Date _2-22-03_

CLIENT PROFILE FOR EYEBROW ENHANCEMENT SERVICES

Name: _____ Date: _____

1. Face Shape: ❑ Round ❑ Long ❑ Square ❑ Oval ❑ Inverted Triangle or Heart ❑ Pear
   ❑ Diamond ❑ Hexagon

2. Circle zone(s) that is/are wide. Upper Middle Lower

3. Circle zone(s) that is/are long. Upper Middle Lower

4. Indicate client's eye set. Close Well Wide

5. Overall size of features: Small Medium Large

6. Size of nose _____

7. Is lip width proportionate to eye width? ❑ yes ❑ no

8. Eye orientation: Almond Even Drooping

9. Color tone: Warm Cool

10. Personality type: ❑ Natural ❑ Conservative ❑ Artistic ❑ Extravagant
    ❑ Relaxed/carefree ❑ Intense ❑ Demure ❑ Other

11. Age group: ❑ Twenties ❑ Thirties ❑ Forties ❑ Fifties ❑ Sixties or older

12. Type of work _____

13. Current condition of eyebrows

    _____

    _____

14. What features would the client like to cosmetically enhance?

    _____

    _____

15. Ideal length of eyebrow: ❑ 1^7/$_8$" ❑ 2" ☑ 2^1/$_8$" ❑ 2^3/$_8$" ❑ other

16. Other important information

    _____

    _____

    _____

    _____

CLIENT PROFILE FOR EYEBROW ENHANCEMENT SERVICES

Name: Rosanna Stanfa   Date: 2-22-03

1. Face Shape: ☐ Round ☐ Long ☐ Square ☑ Oval ☐ Inverted Triangle or Heart ☐ Pear
   ☐ Diamond ☐ Hexagon

2. Circle zone(s) that is/are wide.   (Upper) _slightly_ Middle   Lower

3. Circle zone(s) that is/are long.   Upper   Middle   Lower

4. Indicate client's eye set.   Close   (Well)   Wide

5. Overall size of features: Small   (Medium)   Large w/large eyes

6. Size of nose medium

7. Is lip width proportionate to eye width? ☑ yes ☐ no

8. Eye orientation: (Almond to Even)   Drooping

9. Color tone: (Warm)   Cool

10. Personality type: ☐ Natural ☐ Conservative ☑ Artistic ☐ Extravagant
    ☑ Relaxed/carefree ☐ Intense ☐ Demure ☐ Other

11. Age group: ☑ Twenties ☐ Thirties ☐ Forties ☐ Fifties ☐ Sixties or older

12. Type of work Customer service/student

13. Current condition of eyebrows
    Sparse; needs shape improvement

14. What features would the client like to cosmetically enhance?
    The client would like the illusion of a smaller nose. A brow shape with the appropriate thickness, with symmetry, and that extends to the correct ending point will improve the appearance of the nose.

15. Ideal length of eyebrow: ☐ 1⁷⁄₈" ☐ 2" ☑ 2¹⁄₈" ☐ 2³⁄₈" ☐ other

16. Other important information
    Although client would like thicker brows, she is uncomfortable with a more thickly filled-in look. The client has medium features and large, beautiful eyes. Therefore a medium thickness eyebrow would be the most flattering. However, because of her youthful age and appearance, Rosanna looks wonderful in a thin brow shape, as well.

Name: Rosanna Stanfa   Date: 2-22-03

EYEBROW PRESCRIPTION FORM

In order to maintain beautiful, symmetrical eyebrows, the following items are recommended:

☐ Eyebrow brush/comb

☑ Tweezers

☑ Brow setting product

☑ Eyebrow powder in <u>Dark brown, medium brown, auburn</u> colors

☑ Eyebrow pencil in <u>Dark brown, auburn</u> colors

☑ Eyebrow powder applicator <u>Stiff</u>

☑ Template in <u>2 1/8" length; thin or medium thickness; classic shape</u> shape

☐ Brow perfecting strips in _____ shape

☐ It is recommended that the client have <u>tweezing or waxing</u> (type of hair removal) performed every <u>3-4</u> weeks.

You can schedule your next appointment before leaving today. We will call you to confirm.

(Your Salon Name)

(Salon Telephone Number)

Before

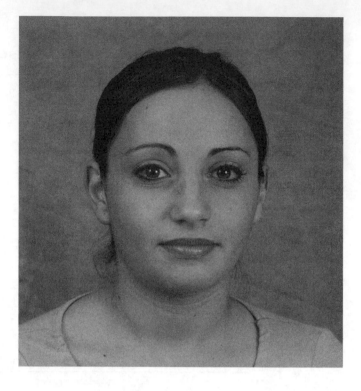

After

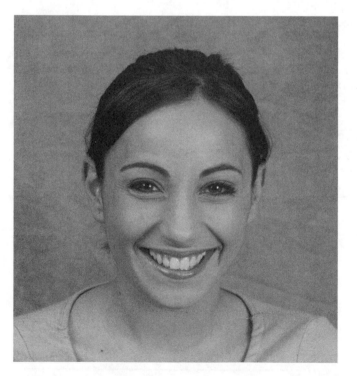

Instructions for Case Study #4

This is your opportunity to design the eyebrows for a client (Figure 13–1).

First, study the features and eyebrows of the client and complete her client profile (Figure 13–3). Use the information provided by the client on her eyebrow enhancement question-naire (Figure 13–2) and the information you recorded about her on the client profile to de-sign a beautiful pair of eyebrows. On Figure 13–1, design the client's eyebrows based on your assessments and fill out the eyebrow pre-scription form (Figure 13–4) to complete the process.

CASE STUDY #4:
PRACTICE CLIENT

EYEBROW ENHANCEMENT QUESTIONNAIRE

Client Name: Amanda J. Bates   Date: 02-22-03

A. Your Eyebrows

   1. What do you like about your eyebrows?
      I like the thickness of my eyebrows.

   2. What would you like to change about your eyebrows?
      My eyebrows are too far apart.

B. Your Health and Medications

   3. Have you used Accutane in the last seven years? no

   4. Are you currently using Accutane? no

   5. Are you currently using Retin-A? no   Renova? no

   6. Are you currently taking blood thinners such as Coumadin? no

   7. Do you use any of the following: Salicyclic acid, alphahydroxy acids, enzymes, scrubs, depilatory creams, vitamin C creams? If so, please list and describe your frequency of use.
      No

   8. Do you have: ❑ Diabetes ❑ Cancer ❑ High Blood Pressure ❑ Acne
      ❑ Phlebitis ❑ Autoimmune Diseases such as Lupus ❑ Sunburn

   9. Have you ever had an adverse reaction after hair removal? If yes, specify the type of hair removal and the adverse reaction you had.
      none

   10. Have you been in the sun or in a tanning bed within the last 48 hours? no

C. Your Preferred Method of Hair Removal

   11. What type of hair removal do you wish to have done today? tweezing or waxing

I have answered all of the questions to the best of my knowledge. I understand that the professional may refuse to provide epilation services because of certain health conditions and that it is in my best interest if the service is not provided. I also understand that there may be swelling or irritation in the areas that are waxed or otherwise epilated. This is only a temporary condition.

Client's Signature Amanda J. Bates   Date 02-22-03

CLIENT PROFILE FOR EYEBROW ENHANCEMENT SERVICES

Name: _Amanda Bates_ Date: _2-22-03_

1. Face Shape: ❑ Round ❑ Long ❑ Square ❑ Oval ❑ Inverted Triangle or Heart ❑ Pear
   ❑ Diamond ❑ Hexagon
2. Circle zone(s) that is/are wide. Upper Middle Lower
3. Circle zone(s) that is/are long. Upper Middle Lower
4. Indicate client's eye set. Close Well Wide
5. Overall size of features: Small Medium Large
6. Size of nose _____
7. Is lip width proportionate to eye width? ❑ yes ❑ no
8. Eye orientation: Almond Even Drooping
9. Color tone: Warm Cool
10. Personality type: ❑ Natural ❑ Conservative ❑ Artistic ❑ Extravagant
    ❑ Relaxed/carefree ❑ Intense ❑ Demure ❑ Other
11. Age group: ❑ Twenties ❑ Thirties ❑ Forties ❑ Fifties ❑ Sixties or older
12. Type of work _____
13. Current condition of eyebrows
    _____
    _____
14. What features would the client like to cosmetically enhance?
    _____
    _____
15. Ideal length of eyebrow: ❑ 1$^7/_8$" ❑ 2$^1/_8$" ❑ 2$^3/_8$" ❑ other
16. Other important information
    _____
    _____
    _____
    _____

Name: __Amanda Bates_____ Date: _____

EYEBROW PRESCRIPTION FORM

In order to maintain beautiful, symmetrical eyebrows, the following items are recommended:

❑ Eyebrow brush/comb

❑ Tweezers

❑ Brow setting product

❑ Eyebrow powder in _____ colors

❑ Eyebrow pencil in _____ colors

❑ Eyebrow powder applicator _____

❑ Template in _____ shape

❑ Brow perfecting strips in _____ shape

❑ It is recommended that the client have _____ (type of hair removal) performed every _____ weeks.

You can schedule your next appointment before leaving today. We will call you to confirm.

(Your Salon Name)

(Salon Telephone Number)

You design the eyebrows
for this client.

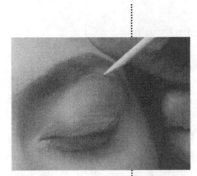

Appendix A

ANSWERS TO CHAPTER QUIZZES

Chapter Two—The Facial Zones and Symmetry

1. a. more
2. c. imaginary line called the midpoint of the face
3. base of the nose, bottom of the chin
4. hairline, just below the eyebrow at its beginning point
5. just below the eyebrows, base of the nose
6. d. both a and b

Chapter Three—The Four Basic Face Shapes

1. c. long
2. d. oval
3. d. oval
4. a. square

Chapter Three—The Four Additional Face Shapes

1. b. diamond
2. a. heart or inverted triangle
3. c. pear or triangle
4. b. inverted triangle and c. heart
5. d. hexagon
6. Each answer will be different. Ask your teacher to compare your drawing of your face shape on Figure 2–17 to the face shape indicated to confirm the correctness of your answer. If you did not complete Figure 2–17, your teacher can verify the correctness of your answer by visual examination.

Chapter Three—Test of the Eight Different Face Shapes

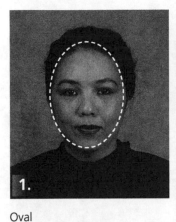

1.

Oval

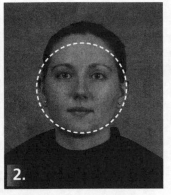

2.

Round

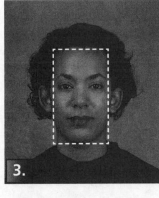

3.

Long

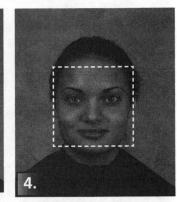

4.

Square

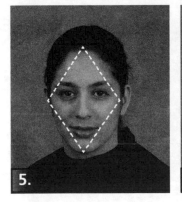

5.

Diamond

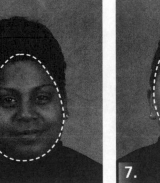

6.

Pear

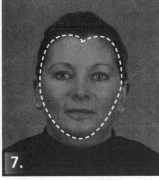

7.

Heart

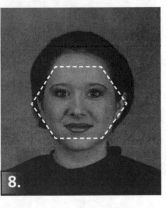

8.

Hexagon

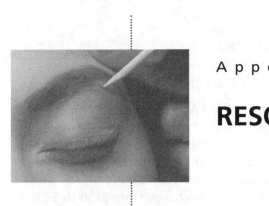

A p p e n d i x   B

RESOURCE DIRECTORY

Hair Removal Training Classes
Provided by the Experts

Waxing Expert

Lori Nestore, CEO
Eva's Esthetics
8201 Capwell Drive
Oakland, CA 94621
(510) 382-0222
www.thewaxqueen.com

Lori Nestore, the "Wax Queen," teaches hands-on eyebrow waxing classes. She is renowned for her Brazilian bikini waxing techniques and videos. A one-day waxing class costs $175. Ms. Nestore is an esthetics, skin care, makeup, and waxing educator at many of the different trade shows and has training videos available for purchase. Contact Betty at Eva's Esthetics at 1 (800) 765-7597 to set up your training or to purchase a videotape.

Threading Expert

Shobha Tummala, CEO
Eyes of the World, Inc. and Shobha™ salon
594 Broadway, Suite 403
New York, NY 10012
(212) 931-8363
www.shobhathreading.com

The Shobha™ Threading Introduction Program (TIP) and customized training programs are currently held at Just Shobha salon in New York City. Because of the increase in demand for this unique hair removal service, Shobha's TIP will soon be accessible in other cities. To discuss your training options, contact Daniel Marein-Efron at (212) 931-8363.

Sugaring Expert

Lina Kennedy, President
Alexandria Professional Body Sugaring™
317 King Street, 2nd Floor
Welland, Ontario
Canada L3B 3K2
1 (800) 957-8427
www.alexandriasugaring.com

To become a certified Alexandria Professional Body Sugaring™ (APBS) practitioner, you must complete both a practical training session and a written examination. To register, contact Alexandria's corporate offices at 1 (800) 957-8427 or at the Web site shown above. The training fees range from $150 to $300.

Laser Expert

Omeed Memar, M.D., Ph.D.
Academic Dermatology & Skin Cancer Institute
30 N. Michigan Avenue, Suite 720
Chicago, IL 60602
(312) 230-0180
www.adsci.com

Dr. Memar holds laser hair removal training classes at his Chicago office. The training program costs $1,500. To set up your laser hair removal training session or to inquire about the program, contact William Brady at (312) 230-0180.

Permanent Makeup Training Classes Provided by the Experts

Permanent Makeup

Rose Marie Beauchemin
The Beau Institute of Permanent & Corrective Cosmetics
2000 Academy Drive, Suite 400
Mt. Laurel, NJ 08054
1 (888) 763-2328
www.beauinstitute.com

At The Beau Institute, you can receive certification in permanent cosmetics (micropigmentation). The Beau Institute program is approved by the American Academy of Micropigmentation (AAM) and the Society of Permanent Cosmetic Professionals (SPCP).

The primary training class is an intensive five-day training session that will teach you how to utilize all different types of equipment and provides comprehensive training in color theory. The primary training class is limited to four students per session and the cost is $3,900. The Beau Institute also offers advanced training classes in different cities. Contact Suzanne at 1 (888) 763-2328 to register for your approved permanent cosmetics training class.

Permanent Makeup

Norma Olivera
Charme International
P.O. Box 38
Miami, FL 33144-0038
1 (888) 242-7631
www.charme1.com (Note: The "1" is the numeral one)

Charme International offers professional permanent makeup training in both basic and advanced formats. The length of training and the cost varies per location and is priced according to the program selected. Classes are held monthly in Miami and in other cities on demand. To schedule your training class, call 1 (888) 242-7631.

Electrolysis

International Guild of Professional Electrologists
202 Boulevard Street, Suite B
High Point, SC 27262
1 (800) 830-3247

Laser

For information regarding laser hair removal, contact:

The American Society for Laser Medicine and Surgery at (715) 845-9283 or log onto their Web site at www.aslms.org

Society of Clinical and Medical Hair Removal Specialists at (608) 831-8009 or at their Web site, www.scmhr.org

Cold Wax Bands

Charme International, 1 (888) 242-7631 or www.charme1.com

Ice Globes (Derm-a-Globe)

Universal Companies, Inc. at 1 (800) 558-5571 or www.universalcompanies.com

Razor Eyebrow Hair Removal

Touch'n Brow at 1 (800) 835-8844

Waxing Products

Amber Products
Ten Chiri Lane
Imperial, PA 15126
1 (800) 821-9188

Cirepil: Shima American Corporation
1961 Concourse Drive, Suite E
San Jose, CA 95131
1 (800) 947-2314, www.cirepilwax.com

Satin Smooth
1 (800) 726-4202
www.satinsmooth.com

Industry Magazines

American Salon
One Park Avenue
New York, NY   10016
(212) 951-6600
www.americansalonmag.com

Beauty Beat
Canadian Hairdresser Magazine
11 Spadina Road
Toronto, Ontario M4R 2S9
(416) 923-1111

DaySpa
628 Densmore Avenue
Van Nuys, CA   91406
(818) 782-7328
www.dayspamagazine.com

Dermascope
2611 N. Belt Line Road, Suite 1017
Sunnyvale, TX   75182
(972) 226-2309
www.dermascope.com

les nouvelles esthetiques
3929 Ponce de Leon Boulevard
Coral Gables, FL   33134
1 (800) 471-0229
www.lneonline.com

Make Up Artist
P.O. Box 4316
Sunland, CA   91041-4316
(818) 504-6770
www.makeupmag.com

Modern Salon/Salon Today
P.O. Box 1414
Lincolnshire, IL 60069
(847) 634-2600
www.modernsalon.com

SalonSENSE
www.salonsense.com

Shades of Beauty
7500 Old Oak Boulevard
Cleveland, OH 44130
1 (888) 527-7008
www.advanstar.com

Skin, Inc.
362 South Schmale Road
Carol Stream, IL 60188-2787
(630) 653-2155
www.SkinInc.com

List of Helpful Web sites

The following are Web sites of professional associations in the beauty industry. They are excellent sources for trade shows, books, and other valuable information.

Aesthetics' International Association
www.aiathekey@aol.com

American Beauty Association
www.abbies.org

American Health and Beauty Aids Inst.
www.ahbai.org

Beauty and Barber Supply Institute, Inc.
www.bbsi.org

Cosmetic, Toiletry & Fragrance Association
www.ctga.org/

Cosmetologists Chicago
www.isnow.com

Day Spa Association
www.dayspaassociation.com

Independent Manufacturers & Dist. Assoc.
www.icmad.org

National Beauty Culturists League
www.nbcl.net

National Coalition of Esthetic & Professional
Association
www.ncea.tv

National Cosmetology Association
www.salonprofessionals.org

Professional Beauty Federation
www.probeautyfederation.org

Society for Permanent Cosmetic Professionals
www.spcp.org

Society of Clinical & Medical Hair Removal
www.scmhr.org

Society of Plastic Surgical Skin Care Specialists
www.surgery.org/

Make-Up Artist magazine Web sites:

On-line source for beauty information
www.makeup411.com

On-line makeup artistry bookstore
www.makeupbooks.com

*PCI—The Medical Journal for Skin Care
Professionals*
www.pcijournal.com

To purchase templates or any other eyebrow
design products, contact:

Adriel, Inc.
1 (800) 273-7126
www.perfectbrow.com

"t" indicates a table on that page.

A

"ABC of Eyebrow Design," 12
Aging
    analysis, effects of aging, 39–40
    corrective techniques to counter effects of,
      73–74
    differences, 3
Altered, asymmetrical eyebrows, 2
Anderson, Pamela, 42
Angres, Gioro, 127
Applicators, for eyebrow powders, 8
Arch
    area, 48
    corrective techniques, 72–73
    shape, 57
Artistic eyebrow shape, 74
Asymmetrical eyebrows, 2
Aucoin, Kevyn, 42

B

Baker, Rick, 18
Beauchemin, Rose Marie, 126–128, 164–165
Beautiful Brows, 2
Beginning point, 56–57
    practice worksheet, 62
Blend electrolysis, 120
Board of Cosmetology, 6
Bobbi Brown Beauty, 4, 22
Brown, Bobbi, 2, 4
Brush, eyebrow, 6–7
Brush test, 47

C

Care-free eyebrow shape, 74
Case studies, 134–158
    full eyebrows, 141–146
      before and after, 146
      client profile, 144
      eyebrow enhancement questionnaire, 142
      eyebrow prescription form, 145
    poorly shaped eyebrows, 147–158
      before and after, 152

      client profile, 150
      eyebrow enhancement questionnaire, 148
      eyebrow prescription form, 151
    practice client
      before and after, 158
      client profile, 156
      eyebrow enhancement questionnaire, 155
      eyebrow prescription form, 157
    sparse eyebrows, 135–140
      before and after, 140
      client profile, 138
      eyebrow enhancement questionnaire, 136
      eyebrow prescription form, 139
Chin
    analysis of, 38–39
    corrective techniques, 71
Client consultation, 84
Close-set eyes, 31
    corrective techniques, 69
Cold wax bands, Web site, 165
Color of brow hair, 48–51
    fill-in suggestions, 50t
Comb, eyebrow, 6–7
Conservative eyebrow shape, 74
Consultation, client, 84
    forms, 84–87
Contraindications
    sugaring, hair removal, 116
    waxing, 105–106t
Corrective techniques, 67–75
    affecting overall style, 74
    to counter effects of age, 73–74
    forehead breadth and overall facial
      appearance, 72–73
    to improve eye set, 68–69
    to improve eye size and orientation, 69–71
    to improve nose appearance, 71
    lips and chin, 71
    in respect to hairstyle, 73
Cosmetic Therapist (CT), 120
Cream, 9

D

Demure eyebrow shape, 74
Derm-a-Globe, 165
Design and enhancement, 78–81, 83–99
  approaches to eyebrow enhancement, 79–81
  client consultation, 84
  client profile, 86
  consultation forms, 84–87
  create a separate fee for, 5
  defined, 4
  eyebrow prescription form, 87
  focusing on, 4–5
  methods
    freehand, 94
      advantages, 78t
      disdvantages, 79t
      step-by-step procedure, 95–96
    template/strip, 88–94
      advantages, 78t
      client preparation, 88
      disadvantages, 79t
      eyebrow shape selection, 90t
      hair removal using brow perfecting strip as
        guide, 93–94
      hair removal using template/brow powder as
        fill-in, 92
      room setup, 88
      step-by-step procedure, 89–91
      tools and supplies, 88
    practice sheets, 97–99
    questionnaire, 85
    tools, 83
    vs. "wax job," 5
Diamond-shaped face, 23–24
  optimal eyebrow shape, 81t
Drooping eye, corrective technique, 70–71

E

Electrolysis, hair removal, 120
  advantages and disadvantages of, 122t
  comparison with other methods, 120t
  training classes for, 165
Ending point, 57–58
  open or closed, 60–61
  practice worksheet, 63
Ethnic differences, 3
Extravagant eyebrow shape, 74
Eyebrow, assessing, 45–54, 46t

color of brow hair, 48–51
  fill-in suggestions, 50t
eyebrow hair, tuft and stubble, 51–52
length, 46–47
practice sheet, 53
texture and growth pattern, 47–48
tinting, 48
tools, 45
Eyebrow brush/comb, 6–7
Eye set, 29–33
  analysis of, 37
  close-set eyes, 31
  corrective techniques, 68–69
  determining
    primary measurement, 30–31
    secondary consideration, 31–32
  one-eye or 3.5 cm. rule, 30
  practice sheet, 33
  proportions of the nose and lips, 32
  tools, 29
Eye size and orientation
  analysis of, 37
  corrective techniques, 69–71

F

Face shapes
  chart, 25
  importance of studying, 20
  quiz, 26–27
    answers, 160–161
  summary, 27
  types of
    diamond-shaped, 23–24
    heart or inverted triangle, 23
    hexagonal-shaped, 24
    long, 21
    no face shapes, 20–21
    oval, 21
    pear-shaped, 24
    round, 22
    square, 21–22
Facial features, 35–44
  analysis of
    effects of age, 39–40
    eye set, 37
    eye size and orientation, 37
    forehead and chin, 38–39
    hairstyle, 39

lips, 38
    nose, 38
    overall feature size, 40–41
    overall style or personality type, 40
breaking the rules, 41–42
corrective techniques, 72–73
tools, 35
worksheet, 43–44
Facial zones, 11–18
    corrective techniques based on length and
        width, 16, 18
    importance of symmetry, 12–13
    measuring, 13–16
    practice exercise, 16
    quiz, 18
        answers, 160
    the three zones, 13
    tools needed, 11
Feature size, overall analysis of, 40–41
Fees, eyebrow design, 5
Fingertip test, 47
Forehead
    analysis of, 38–39
    breadth, corrective techniques, 72–73
Forms, client consultation, 84–87
    client profile, 86
    design and enhancement questionnaire, 85
    eyebrow prescription form, 87
Freehand design methods, 94
    advantages, 78t
    disadvantages, 79t
    step-by-step procedure, 95–96
Full eyebrows, case study, 141–146
    before and after, 146
    client profile, 144
    eyebrow enhancement questionnaire, 142
    eyebrow prescription form, 145

G
Galvanic electrolysis, 120
Gel, 9
Growth pattern of eyebrow, assessing, 47–48

H
Hair
    eyebrow, assessing, 51–52
    structure of, 102
Hair removal, 102–123

challenges for, 102
classification, 102–103
methods
    advantages and disadvantages of each, 122t
    comparison of, 121t
    electrolysis, 120
    laser hair removal, 118–120
    sugaring, 113–116
    threading, 116–118
    tweezing, 103–104
    wax bands, 113
    waxing, 104–112
        contraindications, 105–106t
        soft (strip) wax procedure, 107–112
        technique, 104–105
        types of waxes, 104
    training classes for, 164
Hairstyle, analysis of, 39
Handwashing, 6
Heart shaped face, 23
    optimal eyebrow shape, 81t
Hexagonal–shaped face, 24
    optimal eyebrow shape, 81t

I
Ice Globes, Web site, 165
Ingrown hairs, 104
Intense eyebrow shape, 74
Inverted triangle-shaped face, 23
    optimal eyebrow shape, 81t

K
Kennedy, Lina, 113–114, 164

L
Laser hair removal, 118–120
    advantages and disadvantages of, 122t
    comparison with other methods, 120t
    training classes for, 164, 165
Length of eyebrow, 59–60, 60t
    assessing, 46–47
Lips
    analysis of, 38
    corrective techniques, 71
    determining proportions of, 32
Long face shape, 21
    optimal eyebrow shape, 80t

M

Magazines, Industry, 166
Makeup. *See* Permanent makeup
Making Faces, 42
Making Up, 4
Measuring
    eye set, 30–32
    facial zones, 13–16
Memar, Omeed M., 118–120, 164

N

Natural, unaltered eyebrows, 2, 74
Nd-Yag laser hair removal system, 119
Nelson, Dennis, 6
Nestore, Lori, 104, 164
Nippers, 7
Nose
    analysis of, 38
    determining proportions of, 32
    techniques to improve appearance of,
        71

O

Occupational Safety and Health Administration
    (OSHA), 6
Olivera, Antonio, 113
Olivera, Norma, 165
One-eye or 3.5 cm. rule, 30
    Oprah Magazine, The, 4
OSHA, 6
Oval face shape, 21
    optimal eyebrow shape, 80t

P

Parker, Nancy, 2
Pear-shaped face, 24
    optimal eyebrow shape, 81t
Pencils, 8–9
    vs. powders, 51
Perfecting strips, 10
Permanent makeup, 126–128
    equipment, 127
    evolvement of, 126–127
    preprocedure consultation, 127
    procedure, 127–128
    sanitation, 127
    supplies, 127
    training classes for, 164–165

Personality type
    analysis of, 40
    shapes consistent with, 74
Poorly shaped eyebrows, case study, 147–158
    before and after, 152
    client profile, 150
    eyebrow enhancement questionnaire, 148
    eyebrow prescription form, 151
Powders, eyebrow, 7–8
    black, 50
    brush applicators, 8
    procedure for tinting, 129–132
    taupe, 50
    vs. pencils, 51
Practice client
    before and after, 158
    client profile, 156
    eyebrow enhancement questionnaire, 155
    eyebrow prescription form, 157

R

Razor eyebrow hair removal, 165
Relaxed eyebrow shape, 74
Rex, 4
Round face shape, 22
    optimal eyebrow shape, 80t
Ruler or measuring device, 7

S

Safety and Health in the Salon, 6
Salon Sanitation Rules and Regulations, 6
Sanitation considerations
    brow gel or cream, 9
    brow perfecting strips, 10
    brush applicators, 8
    eyebrow brush/comb, 6–7
    eyebrow pencils, 8–9
    eyebrow powders, 8
    permanent makeup, 127
    powder applicators, 8
    ruler or measuring device, 7
    scissors or nippers, 7
    templates, 9
    tweezers, 7
Scissors or nippers, 7
Shape
    arched vs. rounded, 58–59
    consistent with personality types, 74

elements of
  the arch, 57
    beginning point, 56–57
    ending point, 57–58
  eyebrow length, 59–60, 60t
  open or closed ending point, 60–61
  practice worksheet
    beginning point, 62
    ending point, 63
    using six brow elements, 64
  tools, 55
Smith, Dick, 16, 18
Soare, Anastasia, 12–13
Sparse eyebrows, case study, 135–140
  before and after, 140
  client profile, 138
  eyebrow enhancement questionnaire, 136
  eyebrow prescription form, 139
Square face shape, 21–22
  optimal eyebrow shape, 80t
Stubble hair, 51–52
Style
  analysis of, 40
  corrective techniques that affect overall style, 74
Sugaring, hair removal, 113–116
  advantages and disadvantages of, 122t
  comparison with other methods, 120t
  contraindications, 116
  training classes for, 164
Symmetrical eyebrows, 1–18
  age differences, 3
  altered, asymmetrical eyebrows, 2
  ethnic differences, 3
  focus on eyebrow design, 4–5
  losing fear, gaining confidence, 3–4
  natural, unaltered eyebrows, 2
  quiz, 18
    answers, 160
  symmetry
    defined, 12
    of the face, 12–13
  tools of the trade, 6–10

T
Taupe, fill-in color, 50
Templates, 9
Template/strip design methods, 88–94
  advantages, 78t

choice for eyebrow shape selection, 90t
client preparation, 88
disadvantages, 79t
hair removal using brow perfecting strip as
  guide, 93–94
hair removal using template/brow powder as
  fill-in, 92
room setup, 88
step-by-step procedure, 89–91
tools and supplies, 88
Texture and growth pattern, assessing, 47–48
Thermolysis, 120
Thomson, Rhonda G., 103
Threading, hair removal, 116–118
  advantages and disadvantages of, 122t
  comparison with other methods, 120t
  training classes for, 164
3.5 cm. rule, 30
Tilbury, Charlotte, 4
Tinting eyebrows, 48, 129–132
  assessing, 48
  list of supplies, 130
  procedure, 131–132
  regulations against, 129
  setup for the procedure, 130
Tools of the brow trade, 6–10
  brow gel or cream, 9
  brow perfecting strips, 10
  brush applicator, 8
  eyebrow brush/comb, 6–7
  eyebrow pencils, 8–9
  eyebrow powders, 7–8
  powder applicators, 8
  ruler or measuring device, 7
  scissors or nippers, 7
  templates, 9
  tweezers, 7
Tuft hair, 51–52
Tummala, Shobha, 116–117, 164
Tweezers, 7
Tweezing, hair removal, 103–104
  advantages and disadvantages of, 122t
  comparison with other methods, 121t

W
Wallace, Karen, 129
Waxing, hair removal, 104–112
  advantages and disadvantages of, 122t

Waxing, hair removal *(continued)*
   checklist of supplies, 107
Waxing, hair removal *(continued)*
   comparison with other methods, 120t
   contraindications, 105–106t
   set-up checklist, 108
   soft (strip) wax procedure, 107–112
   soft wax procedure, 100–112
   technique, 104–105
   training classes for, 164

   types of waxes, 104
   wax bands, 113, 165
Waxing products, 165
Web sites, 166–167
Wells, Reggie, 41
Well-set eyes, 31
Westmore, Marvin, 12
Wide-set eyes, 31
   corrective techniques, 68